Recovery and Wellness: Models of Hope and Empowerment for People with Mental Illness

Recovery and Wellness: Models of Hope and Empowerment for People with Mental Illness has been co-published simultaneously as *Occupational Therapy in Mental Health*, Volume 17, Numbers 3/4 2001.

Recovery and Wellness: Models of Hope and Empowerment for People with Mental Illness

Catana Brown, PhD, OTR, FAOTA
Editor

Recovery and Wellness: Models of Hope and Empowerment for People with Mental Illness has been co-published simultaneously as *Occupational Therapy in Mental Health*, Volume 17, Numbers 3/4 2001.

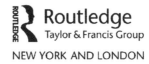

Routledge
Taylor & Francis Group

NEW YORK AND LONDON

Recovery and Wellness: Models of Hope and Empowerment for People with Mental Illness has been co-published simultaneously as *Occupational Therapy in Mental Health*™, Volume 17, Numbers 3/4 2001.

First Published by

The Haworth Press, Inc., 10 Alice Street, Binghamton, NY 13904-1580

Transferred to Digital Printing 2010 by Routledge
270 Madison Ave, New York NY 10016
2 Park Square, Milton Park, Abingdon, Oxon, OX14 4RN

The development, preparation, and publication of this work has been undertaken with great care. However, the publisher, employees, editors, and agents of The Haworth Press and all imprints of The Haworth Press, Inc., including The Haworth Medical Press® and Pharmaceutical Products Press®, are not responsible for any errors contained herein or for consequences that may ensue from use of materials or information contained in this work. Opinions expressed by the author(s) are not necessarily those of The Haworth Press, Inc. With regard to case studies, identities and circumstances of individuals discussed herein have been changed to protect confidentiality. Any resemblance to actual persons, living or dead, is entirely coincidental.

Cover design by Thomas J. Mayshock Jr.

Library of Congress Cataloging-in-Publication Data

Recovery and wellness : models of hope and empowerment for people with mental illness / Catana Brown, editor.
     p. cm.
Co-published simultaneously as Occupational therapy in mental health, vol. 17, nos. 3/4 2001.
Includes bibliographical references and index.
     ISBN 0-7890-1904-3 (hbk. : alk. paper) – ISBN 0-7890-1905-1 (pbk. : alk. paper)
     1. Mentally ill–Rehabilitation. 2. Occupational therapy. 3. Mental health. I. Brown, Catana.
II. Occupational therapy in mental health.
RC439.5 .R4225 2002
616.89′03–dc21

2002008456

Recovery and Wellness: Models of Hope and Empowerment for People with Mental Illness

CONTENTS

PART THREE: APPLICATION OF RECOVERY PRINCIPLES

ABOUT THE EDITOR

Catana Brown, PhD, OTR, FAOTA, received her BS in occupational therapy from Colorado State University, her MA in occupational therapy from New York University, and her PhD in educational psychology and research from the University of Kansas. She is Associate Professor at the University of Kansas Medical Center. Her primary research and practice interests are related to enhancing community living for people with psychiatric disabilities. Together with Edna Hamera and Melisa Rempfer, Dr. Brown has developed a research program examining the impact of person-environment interactions for people with psychiatric disabilities engaging in independent living activities. In collaboration with Winnie Dunn, Dr. Brown has developed the Adult Sensory Profile as a measure of sensory processing preferences. The Adult Sensory Profile provides information that allows individuals to recognize environments that support and inhibit successful and satisfying living. Dr. Brown finds that the principles of wellness and recovery challenge mental health service providers to reenvision their practice to recognize the perspective of the consumer as most important and change the focus of outcomes to empowerment, hope, and successful, satisfying living.

Introduction:
Recovery and Wellness:
Models of Hope and Empowerment
for People with Mental Illness

This volume, *Recovery and Wellness: Models of Hope and Empowerment for People with Mental Illness*, is intended to provide perspective, thought provoking commentary, and practical information. The Recovery Model has emerged from the consumer movement. As discussed in more detail in this collection, the Recovery Model includes the process of gaining control over one's life, appreciating and valuing the uniqueness of oneself, belonging and participating in a community and establishing and realizing hopes and dreams. For many reasons, the philosophy and practices of recovery may be unnerving to service providers. For instance, when one has operated from a position of control, it can be hard to give it up. Service providers may feel that their training and expertise is no longer valued. Furthermore, it can be difficult for service providers to come to terms with their own participation in oppressive systems. On the other hand, as this collection attests, when service providers such as occupational therapists adopt a Recovery Model approach the experience can inspire and enhance the therapist/consumer relationship as well as the therapy process.

Part One of this volume is the consumer's voice. As the editor for this topic, I feel somewhat like an imposter to be presenting concepts, beliefs and practices that come from the experience of living with a mental illness. Therefore the consumer voice assumes a prominent position in this issue. Pat Deegan, a founder of the National Empowerment Center

[Haworth co-indexing entry note]: "Introduction: Recovery and Wellness: Models of Hope and Empowerment for People with Mental Illness." Brown, Catana. Co-published simultaneously in *Occupational Therapy in Mental Health* (The Haworth Press, Inc.) Vol. 17, No. 3/4, 2001, pp. 1-3; and: *Recovery and Wellness: Models of Hope and Empowerment for People with Mental Illness* (ed: Catana Brown) The Haworth Press, Inc., 2001, pp. 1-3. Single or multiple copies of this article are available for a fee from The Haworth Document Delivery Service [1-800-HAWORTH, 9:00 a.m. - 5:00 p.m. (EST). E-mail address: getinfo@haworthpressinc.com].

1

and leading author on recovery, opens the issue with a first-person account of her experience of recovering from schizophrenia. She also provides suggestions for ways in which service providers can support recovery. This is followed by another first person account by Cherie Bledsoe who discusses the experience of being a consumer provider. Her paper outlines both the challenges and triumphs as one of the first consumer providers in a mental health center. Part One ends with Susan Mack's account of growing up with a mental illness, becoming an occupational therapist and discovering the meaning of recovery.

Part Two includes two papers with a philosophical perspective. Juli McGruder discusses the problems inherent in the medicalization of mental illness. She presents an interesting counter argument to current efforts aimed at destigmatizing mental illness by presenting it as a biological disease. René Padilla is equally provocative in presenting three approaches to occupational therapy psychoeduction. He argues for a liberationist approach in which the teacher acts as model, learning along with the student.

Part Three ends the publication with four papers focusing on the application of recovery principles. Jason Wollenberg presents an overview of the occupational therapy process within a recovery framework. From referral to the discontinuation of therapy, recovery impacts the way in which services are delivered. My contribution to the volume falls in this section. In a fairly specific application piece, understanding sensory processing and designing environments to support particular preferences is discussed. Mary Ellen Copeland presents her Wellness Recovery Action Plan. This plan, now used by many with long term illnesses, provides a system for integrating coping and wellness strategies into everyday life. The volume ends with an application to research. Melisa Rempfer and Jill Knott present Participatory Action Research as a model of establishing partnerships between researchers and consumers. They provide specific application, examples and benefits for this approach in research related to psychiatric disabilities.

It is my hope that occupational therapists will find this collection both interesting and stimulating, that the ideas and applications will lead to changes in practice. The inherent optimism of occupational therapists is clearly compatible with recovery. Let us share in the hopes and dreams of recovery.

ACKNOWLEDGMENTS

First, I would like to thank all of the contributors to this volume. Their work is what makes it special. In addition, I would like to thank Mary Donohue for the opportunity to put this project together. I would like to thank the staff and consumers at the Wyandot Center for teaching me, both through words and actions, what recovery is all about. Finally, I would like to acknowledge all of the people who have written, talked about, lived and embarked upon the recovery experience.

Catana Brown, PhD, OTR, FAOTA

PART ONE:
CONSUMER/SURVIVOR PERSPECTIVES

Recovery as a Self-Directed Process of Healing and Transformation

Patricia E. Deegan, PhD

SUMMARY. This paper describes a first person account of recovering from schizophrenia. Recovery is described as a transformative process as opposed to merely achieving stabilization or returning to baseline. The self-directed nature of the recovery process is highlighted with suggestions as to how professionals can support recovery. *[Article copies available for a fee from The Haworth Document Delivery Service: 1-800-HAWORTH. E-mail address: <getinfo@haworthpressinc.com> Website: <http://www.HaworthPress.com> © 2001 by The Haworth Press, Inc. All rights reserved.]*

KEYWORDS. Recovery, schizophrenia, self-help, coping, hope

Patricia E. Deegan is a co-founder of the Boston University Institute for the Study of Human Resilience and Senior Director of the Joshua Tree Center for Ex-Patient Studies.

[Haworth co-indexing entry note]: "Recovery as a Self-Directed Process of Healing and Transformation." Deegan, Patricia E. Co-published simultaneously in *Occupational Therapy in Mental Health* (The Haworth Press, Inc.) Vol. 17, No. 3/4, 2001, pp. 5-21; and: *Recovery and Wellness: Models of Hope and Empowerment for People with Mental Illness* (ed: Catana Brown) The Haworth Press, Inc., 2001, pp. 5-21. Single or multiple copies of this article are available for a fee from The Haworth Document Delivery Service [1-800-HAWORTH, 9:00 a.m. - 5:00 p.m. (EST). E-mail address: getinfo@haworthpressinc.com].

Recovery is often defined conservatively as returning to a stable baseline or former level of functioning. However, many people, including myself, have experienced recovery as a transformative process in which the old self is gradually let go of and a new sense of self emerges. In this paper I will share my personal experience of recovery as a self-directed process of healing and transformation and offer some suggestions as to how professionals can support the recovery process.

When I was seventeen years old and a senior in high school, I began to have experiences of severe emotional distress that eventually were labeled as mental illness. Illustration 1 symbolizes how I experienced myself and how others perceived me before I was diagnosed with schizophrenia.

The most immediate impression of this symbolic flower is its integrity and wholeness. This represents the fact that before being diagnosed with mental illness there was a basic congruity between how I understood myself and how others perceived me. In addition, each of the petals on the flower represent aspects of who I was. I was the oldest child in

ILLUSTRATION 1. How I Was Seen by Others and Understood Myself Before Being Diagnosed with Mental Illness

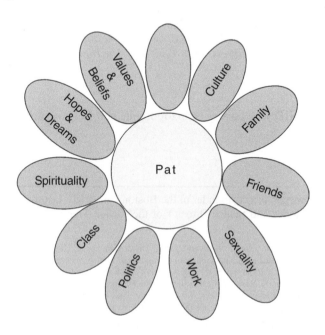

a large working-class Irish Catholic family. My friends, my social role as a worker and student, my spirituality, values and beliefs, culture, family and socio-economic class all converged to form the unique individual I was at seventeen years old.

Notice that one of the petals on the flower is empty. This empty petal symbolizes the idea that my life opened onto a future. That future was unknown and ambiguous. It was precisely because my future was unknown that I could project my hopes, dreams and aspirations into it. That is, hope arises in relation to an open, ambiguous and uncertain future. As a teenager, I remember my dream was to become a coach for women's athletic teams. I was a gifted athlete and did just enough academic work to get passing grades so I could continue to compete on varsity teams. At seventeen I could not have imagined that someday I would have a doctorate in clinical psychology and be writing a chapter for a book!

The image of me as a whole, unique and promising young person began to crumble during the winter of my seventeenth year. Even now I can vividly recall some aspects of the emotional distress I began to experience. For instance, during basketball practice it became harder and harder to catch a ball. My depth perception and coordination seemed strangely impaired and I found myself being hit in the head with passes rather than catching the ball. Objects around me also began to look very different. Countertops, chairs and tables had a threatening, ominous physiognomy. Everything was thrown into a sharp, angular and frightening geometry. The sense that things had utilitarian value escaped me. For instance, a table was no longer something to rest objects upon. Instead a table became a series of right angles pointing at me in a threatening way.

A similar shift in my perception and understanding occurred when people spoke to me. Language became hard to understand. Gradually I could not understand what people were saying at all. Instead of focusing on words, I focused on the mechanical ways that mouths moved and the way that screwdrivers had taken the place of proper teeth. It became difficult to believe that people were really who they said they were. What I remember most was the extraordinary fear that kept me awake for days and the terrible conviction I was being killed and needed to defend myself.

The adults around me eventually decided that I had "gone crazy," and I soon found myself being escorted up a hospital elevator by two men in white uniforms. Once in the mental hospital, I was diagnosed with schizophrenia. Illustration 2 represents the way I was viewed by those around me once I had been diagnosed:

ILLUSTRATION 2. How I Was Seen by Others After Being Diagnosed with
Mental Illness

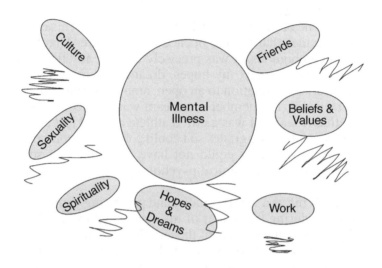

Whereas before being diagnosed I was seen as a whole person, after
being diagnosed it was as if professionals put on a pair of distorted
glasses through which they viewed me as fundamentally ill and broken.
The jagged lines represent the distorted lens through which I was
viewed. It seemed that everything I did was interpreted through the lens
of psychopathology. For instance, when growing up, my grandmother
used to say I had ants-in-my-pants. Now, in a mental hospital, I was agitated. I never cried very much while growing up, but after diagnosis I
was told I had flat affect. I was always quiet, shy, and introverted. Now I
was guarded, suspicious and had autistic features. And in a classic dou-
ble-bind, if I protested these pathologized interpretations of myself then
that was further proof I was schizophrenic because I lacked insight!

Notice also that in the first illustration there was congruity between
how I viewed myself and how others viewed me but after being diagnosed there was a lack of congruity. That is, although I was severely dis-
tressed, I still felt that deep down I was myself–Pat. However, the
professionals, and later my family and friends, seemed to forget about Pat

and were now more interested in "the schizophrenic." This is symbolized by the substitution of a diagnosis for my name in the center circle.

After being diagnosed, mental illness took on a master status in terms of how others viewed me. The fact that I was a unique person with my own spirituality, culture, sexuality, work history, and values and beliefs was secondary–one might even say perfunctory. This is symbolized by the petals being broken off, and even missing altogether. What mattered most to psychiatrists, social workers, nurses, psychologists and occupational therapists was that I *was* a schizophrenic. My identity had been reduced to an illness in the eyes of those who worked with me. It was only a matter of time before I began to internalize this stigmatized and dehumanized view of myself.

Dehumanization is an act of violence, and treating people as if they were illnesses is dehumanizing. Everyone loses when this happens. People, especially people who are feeling very vulnerable, internalize what professionals tell them. People learn to say what professionals say; "I am a schizophrenic, a bi-polar, a borderline, etc." Yet instead of weeping at such a capitulation of personhood, most professionals applaud these rote utterances as "insight." Of course the great danger of reducing a person to an illness is that there is no one left to do the work of recovery. If all professionals see are schizophrenics, borderlines, bi-polars, etc., then the resilient strengths and gifts of the individual are ignored and sacrificed to the gods of the DSM-IV.

Notice that the empty petal is missing from Illustration 2. This symbolizes the fact that because of my diagnosis professionals lost hope that I could have a meaningful future. Recall how in the Illustration 1 the empty petal symbolized the unknown, ambiguous future into which I projected my hopes, dreams and aspirations. Once diagnosed with schizophrenia, professionals acted as if my future and my fate were sealed. I recall the day this happened to me: I asked my psychiatrist what my diagnosis was. He looked at me from behind his desk and said, "Miss Deegan, you have a disease called schizophrenia. Schizophrenia is a disease like diabetes. Just like diabetics have to take medications for the rest of their lives, you will have to take medications for the rest of your life. If you go into this halfway house, I think you will be able to cope."

"YOU ARE WRONG"

Coping is definitely not what a teenager wants to do on a Friday night! I was not at all inspired by the thought of a life spent coping. I remember feeling like I had been hit by a truck upon hearing his words. Then I remember my mind racing, trying to think of one famous person who was diagnosed with schizophrenia. I instinctively needed to identify someone who had beat the odds but nobody came to mind. As the psychiatrist continued to babble on, I felt a surge of anger rising up within me. Although I knew better than to get too angry in a psychiatrist's office, I found the words forming silently inside me: "You are wrong. I'm not a schizophrenic. You are wrong!"

Today I understand that this psychiatrist did not give me a diagnosis. He gave me a prognosis of doom. Essentially this psychiatrist was telling me that by virtue of the diagnosis of schizophrenia, my future was fait accompli. He was telling me that the best I could hope for was to cope and remain on medications for the rest of my life. He was saying my life did not open upon a future that was ambiguous and unknown. He was saying my future was sealed and the book of my life had already been written nearly 100 years earlier by Emil Kraepelin (1912), the psychiatrist who wrote a pessimistic account of schizophrenia that influences psychiatrists even to this day. According to Kraepelin, my life, like the life of all schizophrenics, would be a chronic deteriorating course ending in dementia (Kruger 2000).

It was this prognosis of doom, this life sentence, this death before death that I instinctively rejected when the words "You are wrong" formed silently within me. With the wisdom of hindsight I understand why this moment in the psychiatrist's office was a major turning point in my recovery process. When I rejected the prognosis of doom I simultaneously affirmed my worth and dignity. Through my angry indignation I was affirming that "I am more than that, more than a schizophrenic." Importantly, it was my anger that announced the resurrection of my dignity after it had been so battered down during hospitalizations. My angry indignation was a sign I was alive and well and resilient and intent on fighting for a life that had meaning and hope. What some would have seen as denial and a lack of insight into my illness, I experienced as a turning point in my recovery process.

MY DREAM

Rejecting the hopeless prognosis through angry indignation happened almost like a reflex. And just as quickly as I turned away from the prophecy of doom, I found myself asking–so now what? In other words, I turned away from a hopeless path but also, at the same time, had to turn toward something. What I remember was that when I left the psychiatrist's office, I stood in the hallway and had an image in my mind's eye of a big heavy key chain–the type carried by the most important and powerful professionals who have the keys to all the hospital doors. I found myself thinking, "I'll become Dr. Deegan and I'll make the mental health system work the right way so no one else ever gets hurt in it again." And this plan became what I have come to call my survivor's mission. Yes, it was a grand dream that would have to be molded and modified with time and maturity. But it was my dream nonetheless and it became the project around which I organized my recovery.

I did not tell anyone about my dream. In hindsight this was very wise. Imagine if I had gone to my treatment team as an 18-year-old girl diagnosed with chronic schizophrenia, having had three hospitalizations, barely graduating from high school with combined SAT scores of under 800–and announcing that my plan was to become Dr. Deegan and transform the mental health system so it helped instead of hurt people. Delusions of grandeur! Clearly it was better to keep my dream to myself.

THE COKE AND SMOKE SYNDROME

I wish I could say that having found a survivor's mission I resolutely marched forward in my recovery. But recovery does not strike like a bolt of lightening wherein one is suddenly and miraculously cured. The truth is, when I returned home after that transformative experience, I proceeded to sit and chain smoke in the same chair I had been sitting and smoking in for months. In other words, although everything had changed within me, nothing had changed on the outside yet. Here is what people would have seen me doing at that time in my life:

I turn my gaze back over the years. I can see her yellow, nicotine-stained fingers. I can see her shuffled, stiff, drugged walk. Her eyes do not dance. The dancer has collapsed and her eyes are dark and they stare endlessly into nowhere . . . She forces herself out of bed at 8 o'clock in the morning. In a drugged haze she sits in a chair, the same chair every day. She is smoking cigarettes. Cigarette after cigarette. Cigarettes mark the passing of time. Cigarettes are proof that time is passing and that fact, at least, is a relief. From 9 a.m. to noon she sits and smokes and stares. Then she has lunch. At 1 p.m. she goes back to bed to sleep until 3 p.m. At that time she returns to the chair and sits and smokes and stares. Then she has dinner. She returns to the chair at 6 p.m. Finally, it is 8 o'clock in the evening, the long-awaited hour, the time to go back to bed and to collapse into a drugged and dreamless sleep.

The same scenario unfolds the next day, and then the next, and then the next, until the months pass by in numbing succession marked only by the next cigarette and then the next . . . (Deegan 1993, p. 8)

For many months I lived in what I came to call the coke and smoke syndrome. The first truly proactive step I took in my recovery process occurred at the prompting of my grandmother. Each day she would come into the living room as I smoked cigarettes. She would ask me if I would like to go food shopping with her and each day I would say "No." She asked only once a day and that made it feel like a real invitation rather than nagging. For reasons I cannot account for, one day after months of sitting and smoking, I said "Yes" to her invitation. I now understand that "yes," and the subsequent trip to the market where I would only push the cart, was the first active step I took in my recovery. Other small steps followed such as making an effort to talk to a friend who had come to visit or going for a short walk.

RECOVERY STRATEGIES

Eventually it was suggested I take a course in English Composition at the local community college and I agreed. Going to college presented me with a whole new set of challenges such as managing anxiety, distressing voices and suspicions during class time as well as finding ways to concentrate in order to do homework. At the time there were no organized self-help and mutual support groups for ex-patients so I was very much on my own in terms of developing coping strategies. Table 1 lists some of the most important self-care strategies I developed.

Through a process of trial and error I discovered self-care strategies that worked for me. For instance, I learned at a young age that street drugs, alcohol and even some over-the-counter drugs such as certain types of cold medications were not good for me. I avoided these and am certain this helped my recovery.

Relationships–especially learning to balance time alone and time with people–have always been an important self-care strategy for me. In the beginning my relationships were quite limited and lopsided in the sense that people tended to care more for me than I did for them. Over

TABLE 1

Some of My Recovery Strategies

- No drugs or alcohol
- Finding tolerant environments
- Relationships
- Spirituality and finding meaning in my suffering
- A sense of purpose and direction; survivor's mission around which to organize my recovery
- Routine
- Day at a time, hour at a time, minutes at a time
- Study, learn, and work
- A willingness to take responsibility for myself and accepting that no one could do the work of recovery for me
- Willingness to do psychotherapy to work through trauma history
- Meeting others in recovery and learning not to be ashamed
- Development of self-care skills:
  - How to avoid delusional thinking
  - How to cope with voices
  - How to cope with anxiety
  - How to rest, pace myself, sleep
  - Prayer, meditation
  - Sensory diet

time I learned to become more intimate with people and to develop more mutually reciprocal relationships.

Routines were important to me, especially in the early years of my recovery. Sometimes when everything was falling apart inside of me, it was good to be able to rely on routines that would give form and structure to the chaos I was experiencing. Having a sense of purpose, a reason to get up in the morning and a goal to organize my recovery around were important. Studying a wide range of subjects, especially world religions, philosophy and archetypal psychology, were helpful in my efforts to make sense of the experiences I was having. My spirituality and faith tradition had always been a resource for me. Spiritual practices and making an effort to have conscious contact with my God became integral to my recovery. My spirituality offered me a way of finding meaning in my suffering, and that in turn helped me through feelings of anguished futility, self pity and the inevitable "Why me?" questions that come with difficult passages.

TOLERANT ENVIRONMENTS

I find that tolerant environments have always been helpful in my recovery. I discovered this quite accidentally when I moved from a single rented room into an apartment I shared with a group of ex-hippies. In that environment my roommates were quite open to all sorts of unusual experiences and their world-view included experiences like auras, astral travel, and the like. In such a tolerant atmosphere my psychotic experiences were not viewed as terribly deviant and nobody overreacted. Instead, people were non-intrusive, generally kind and supportive, and they gave me the room I needed to experience my madness. In this tolerant environment I learned that although psychosis does not come with directional signs and maps, it does have a certain terrain and topography. I found that if one returns to the psychotic landscape over time, one can come to know it, to learn not to fear it, and to master ways to navigate through it. Had I been in a halfway house where one must be almost more normal than normal, I fear I may never have learned these important lessons in my self-care and my recovery may have been slowed or prevented.

TOLERATING DISCOMFORT

Learning to tolerate discomfort, anxiety and symptoms meant developing a new relationship to time. I can remember trying to make it through a one hour class and sometimes watching the clock, repeating to myself, "I can make it just one more minute." Each success built my sense of self-efficacy and confidence in my skills to endure and persevere. Also, I learned to tell myself that "Tomorrow will come." This phrase took on great significance for me in my recovery. Tomorrow will come meant that if today was too painful, it too would pass. The assurance that a new day would dawn–and with it new possibilities–became a great comfort in my recovery.

People often ask me if medications were a significant part of my recovery. I did not find psychiatric drugs to be particularly helpful except for their capacity to help me sleep during very stressful times. I found the emotional numbing, sexual dysfunction, and overall sluggishness caused by the drugs to be more disabling at times than psychotic symptoms. The key for me was learning to use medications in conjunction with self-help strategies and overall self-care practices. The more skilled I became in using self-help, the less I relied on medications.

Later in my recovery I became willing to do psychotherapy in order to work through a history of child abuse. This was long and difficult work, and I am glad I embarked on it after I had established myself in a meaningful career and had a strong network of friends. I needed to be firmly planted in the present as an adult, in order to look back at the trauma in my childhood. In the course of doing the trauma work I sought out the help of an occupational therapist who specialized in sensory defensiveness in adults. She helped me learn a myriad of coping strategies including use of a sand blanket, joint compression, tactile brushing, and the use of a sensory diet to help me modulate sensory input and affective arousal. These strategies have proved tremendously helpful and are a part of my everyday recovery "toolkit."

SELF-HELP STRATEGIES

I developed many self-help strategies that made it possible to cope with a myriad of symptoms. For instance, I learned to use headphones and ear plugs to stop the distressing voices I heard. I learned to avoid certain types of situations and subjects that would lead me into the vortex of delusional thinking. Physical exercise, especially daily walks in the woods, remain an important self-help strategy for me. Overall physical health, a good diet, a willingness to pace myself and to get sleep were all important strategies that I learned and refined over time.

OVERCOMING INTERNALIZED STIGMA

For me recovery meant learning to overcome the shame and stigma I had internalized. Like many people in the early stages of recovery, I saw becoming normal as a goal. I remember going through a phase where I measured my wellness by how little medication I took and how few mental patients I was associated with. In fact, there was a time when I refused to be around people with psychiatric histories. I thought the further I could get away from them, the further I could distance myself from my own history. For many years I settled for simply "passing" as a normal person.

The pressure to remain in the closet about my psychiatric history did not come just from me. There was a good deal of social pressure to keep my psychiatric history a secret. For instance, as a student in graduate school, there was the unspoken rule that if you had a psychiatric history there was no way professors would allow you to become a clinical psychologist. In the 1980s, before passage of the Americans with Disabilities Act, I knew of no professionals who were out about having a psychiatric history and I did not feel comfortable being the first. Therefore I hid my psychiatric history and that meant re-living many traumatic memories with no support. For instance, I remember doing my first internship in a state hospital and on the first day having a panic attack when the heavy metal door slammed shut behind me. I can remember freezing in a type of flashback when I witnessed a person being dragged into restraints. Only a few years ago that had been me! Living in the closet meant I had to work through this part of my professional development alone.

I found living in the closet was the same as living a lie. I grew tired of being ashamed. By the time I had finished my doctorate I began to meet psychiatric survivors and activists who had recovered. Meeting these friends was an epiphany for me. They taught me that it was not my problem that the world insisted I be either a clinical psychologist *or* a mental patient. It was not my problem people insisted I wear one hat or the other in order to make them comfortable. I was a whole person. I was a person with a psychiatric history who was also a clinical psychologist. If the world did not have a category for that, then that was the world's problem, not mine. I did not have to live in the closet so others would feel comfortable. And importantly, I was not alone. There were others like me, and if we supported one another, we could lead our lives with pride. Thus, rejecting internalized stigma and learning not to be ashamed of myself was a big step in my recovery process. Illustration 3 symbolically captures the transformed sense of self I now experience.

RECOVERY AS A PROCESS OF TRANSFORMATION

This illustration symbolizes how I have been transformed through the recovery process. The flower is no longer broken as in Illustration 2. My name rather than my diagnosis has resumed its rightful place at the center of who I am. The empty petal has been restored because I have a future that remains ambiguous and unknown and into which I can project my dreams and aspirations. I have used all of the gifts and resources

ILLUSTRATION 3. Recovery: I Am a Person, Not an Illness

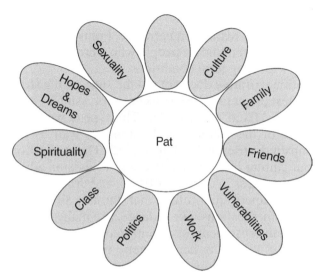

at my disposal to achieve my recovery and so the petals have been restored to the flower.

Notice that one new petal has been added to the flower–vulnerabilities. I do not feel I have a residual mental illness that is in remission and that may get activated at some later time. However, like most people, I live with certain vulnerabilities. I still use my self-care strategies on a daily basis in order to stay well. I am a person, not an illness. I can use what I have learned through my recovery to continue to lead a whole and vibrant life.

Recovery has been a process of healing and transformation for me. I am not the same person I was before I went crazy. My madness has been a kind of fire through which I have walked and through which I have been changed. There were times in the early years when all I wanted was to go back to who I had been. I wanted to go back to high school and pursue that dream of becoming an athletic coach. I wanted to go back and "feel like myself again."

THE RESTITUTION NARRATIVE

This wish to return to the former self is understandable and is called a restitution narrative by Frank (1995). The restitution narrative is a story that some people tell about their recovery. Its basic storyline is: "Yesterday I was healthy, today I am sick, but tomorrow I will be healthy again." The phrases "good as new" and "I feel like myself again" capture the essence of the restitution narrative. Frank notes that restitution narratives are most often told by people who were ill recently, and least often by those with long term conditions.

The restitution narrative does not tell the story of the struggling self, but rather is a testament to the expertise of professionals and their technologies that have "fixed" the problem. This type of narrative is the preferred narrative of the medical professions, as well as the powerful interest groups/industries behind medicine. The restitution narrative permeates our culture in a myriad of ways. Television advertisements, infomercials, brochures in doctors' offices, and drug advertisements in magazines, newspapers and professional journals all tell of the restorative wonders of medications. For instance, in a mainstream psychiatric journal, a 1996 advertisement for an anti-depressant drug shows a little girl with a big smile, racing her energetic mom up the stairs in their home. In bright crayon colors, a note from the child reads: "I got my mommy back." Then comes the name of the drug with the middle letter in bright crayon color. The restitution storyline is clear: Depression came, the medicine worked and then this mom was restored to her family as good as new. Through the power of such images and advertising, the restitution narrative has become a cultural expectation of how all illness should end happily ever after.

For those of us who have struggled for years, the restitution storyline does not hold true. For us, recovery is not about going back to who we were. It is a process of becoming new. It is a process of discovering our limits, but it is also a process of discovering how these limits open upon new possibilities. Transformation, rather than restoration, becomes our path.

TRANSFORMATION PROCESSES

Transformation narratives emphasize the agency of the self in the healing process as opposed to crediting professionals with curative powers. In this light, the task of mental health professionals becomes one of supporting people and helping them build skills and a sense of agency. Helping people learn to become self-directing rather than compliant is a goal of the recovery process.

Because recovery is a unique journey for each individual, there is no cookbook approach. Mental health professionals must explore the special gifts and resources of each individual and help them mobilize these resources in the service of recovery. Begin with asking people what they already do to cope with various distressing symptoms. In this respect the research of Vaughn Carr (1988) is instructive. He asked 200 people diagnosed with schizophrenia to respond to a questionnaire about how they coped with various symptoms. In addition to the coping strategies identified in the questionnaire, nearly half (n = 92) identified other strategies they used. In all, 350 individual coping strategies were identified. Carr concludes that:

> From the foregoing it should appear obvious that schizophrenic patients are not simply passive victims of their illness. On the contrary, these results together with the literature reviewed suggest that in schizophrenia patients can play an active role in the management of their illness, particularly in the containment of its symptoms . . . The experiences of schizophrenia is evidently a learning process in which patients make active attempts to master the illness and not have it dominate them. (p. 350)

People are more than their diagnoses. People diagnosed with mental illness are resilient and are more than passive victims of disease processes. Professionals who learn to collaborate with the active, resilient, adaptive self of the client will find themselves collaborating in new and rewarding ways with people who may have been viewed as hopeless by others who reify diagnoses and related prophecies of doom.

EMPIRICAL EVIDENCE OF RECOVERY

There is hope for recovery. We can no longer justify the pessimism and prophecies of doom that surround diagnoses like schizophrenia. We now have seven long-term studies that ground our hope for recovery in empirical findings (Bleuler 1968, 1974; Tsuang, M.T., Woolson, R.F. and Fleming, J.A. 1979; Ciompi 1980; Huber, Gross, Schuttler and Linz 1980; Harding, C.M., Brooks, G.W., Ashikaga, T., Strauss, J.S., and Breier, A. 1987a, b; Ogawa, K., Miya, M., Watarai, A., Nakazawa, M., Yuasa, S., and Utena, H. 1987; DeSisto, M.J., Harding, C.M., McCormick, R.V., Ashikaga, T. and Gautum, S. 1995a, b). The seven studies were conducted in different countries including the United States, Japan,

Switzerland, and Germany. Each of the seven long term studies have large cohorts of between 140-502 research participants diagnosed with major mental illnesses. The length of study during which the research participants were studied ranged from 22 years-37 years. The recovery rate in these seven long term studies ranged from 46% to 68%. That is, half to two-thirds of people diagnosed with major mental illnesses including schizophrenia were found to show significant or complete recovery over time. Even in the second or third decade after being diagnosed, people still go on to significant or full recovery. We should never lose hope (Harding and Zahniser 1994).

Recovery is not the privilege of a few exceptional clients. We can now tell people the good news that empirical data indicate most people do recover. Because there is no way to predict who will or will not recover, we should approach each person as being able to recover if given sufficient opportunity to build skills and supports. In this way professionals can stop the iatrogenic wounding of hopelessness and begin working with clients on that the transformative journey of recovery.

REFERENCES

Bleuler, M. (1968). A 23-year longitudinal study of 208 schizophrenics and impressions in regard to the nature of schizophrenia. In: *The transmission of schizophrenia* (Eds. D. Rosenthal and S.S. Kety). Oxford: Pergamon Press Ltd., p. 3-12.

Bleuler, M. (1974). The long-term course of the schizophrenic psychoses. *Psychological Medicine*, 4, 244-254.

Carr, V. (1988). Patients' techniques for coping with schizophrenia: An exploratory study. *British Journal of Medical Psychology*, 61, 339-352.

Ciompi, L. (1980). Catamnestic long-term study on the course of life and aging of schizophrenics. *Schizophrenia Bulletin*, 6, 4, 606-618.

Deegan, P.E. (1993). Recovering our sense of value after being labeled mentally ill. *Psychosocial Nursing and Mental Health Services*, *31*, 4, 7-11.

Desisto, M.J., Harding, C.M., McCormick, R.V., Ashikaga, T. & Gautum, S. (1995a). The Maine and Vermont three-decade studies of serious mental illness I. Matched comparison of cross-sectional outcome. *British Journal of Psychiatry*,161, 331-338.

Desisto, M.J., Harding, C.M., McCormick R.V., Ashikaga, T. & Gautum, S. (1995b). The Maine-Vermont three decades study studies of serious mental illness: Longitudinal course of comparisons. *British Journal of Psychiatry*, 167, 338-342.

Frank, A.W. (1995). *The wounded storyteller: Body, illness and ethics*. Chicago: The University of Chicago Press.

Harding, C. M., Brooks, G.W., Ashikaga, T., Strauss, J.S. & Breier, A. (1987a). The Vermont longitudinal study of persons with severe mental illness, I: Methodology, study sample, and overall status 32 years later. *American Journal of Psychiatry*, 144: 6, 718-726.

Harding, C.M., Brooks, G.W., Ashikaga, T., Strauss, J.S., & Breier, A. (1987b). The Vermont longitudinal study of persons with severe mental illness, II: Long-term outcome of subject who retrospectively met DSM-III criteria for schizophrenia. *American Journal of Psychiatry*,144:6, 727-735.

Harding, C.M & Zahniser, J.H. (1994). Empirical correction of seven myths about schizophrenia with implications for treatment. *Acta Psychiatrica Scandinavica, 90*, supplement 384, 140-146.

Huber, G., Gross, G., Schuttler, R. & Linz, M. (1980). Longitudinal studies of schizophrenic patients. *Schizophrenia Bulletin*, 6:4, 592-605.

Kraepelin, E. (1912). *Clinical psychiatry: A textbook for students and physicians.* (Rev. ed. A.R. Diefendorf, Trans.). New York: Macmillan. (Original work published 1883).

Kruger, A. (2000). Schizophrenia: Recovery and Hope. *Psychiatric Rehabilitation Journal*, 24, 2-37.

Ogawa, K., Miya, M., Watarai, A., Nakazawa, M., Yuasa, S., & Utena, H. (1987). *British Journal of Psychiatry*, 151, 758-765.

Tsuang, M.T., Woolson, R.F., & Fleming, J.A. (1979). Long-term outcome of major psychoses 1: Schizophrenia and affective disorders compared with psychiatrically symptom-free surgical conditions. *Archives of General Psychiatry*, 36, 1295-1301.

Unique Eyes
and Different Windows of Opportunity:
The Consumer Provider Perspective

Cherie Bledsoe, PhD

SUMMARY. The writer discusses her personal experiences of being a consumer of mental health services and, at the same time, working as a mental health professional. She includes the challenges and benefits of this experience, as well as the "sparks, pushes, and bumps" of this dual role. Also included are current and future trends of mental health recovery, suggested to be the key to wellness for consumers. *[Article copies available for a fee from The Haworth Document Delivery Service: 1-800-HAWORTH. E-mail address: <getinfo@haworthpressinc.com> Website: <http://www.HaworthPress.com> © 2001 by The Haworth Press, Inc. All rights reserved.]*

KEYWORDS. Consumer provider, recovery, wellness, mental illness, believable hope

Every now and then, my mentor stops me and asks, "Why are you still here?" Once I stop laughing at the question, I remember my story.

Cherie Bledsoe is a Consumer Affairs and Development Specialist at the Wyandot Center for Community Behavioral Health Care in Kansas City, and Executive Director of S.I.D.E., Inc., a consumer-run organization in Wyandotte County, KS.

[Haworth co-indexing entry note]: "Unique Eyes and Different Windows of Opportunity: The Consumer Provider Perspective." Bledsoe, Cherie. Co-published simultaneously in *Occupational Therapy in Mental Health* (The Haworth Press, Inc.) Vol. 17, No. 3/4, 2001, pp. 23-42; and: *Recovery and Wellness: Models of Hope and Empowerment for People with Mental Illness* (ed: Catana Brown) The Haworth Press, Inc., 2001, pp. 23-42. Single or multiple copies of this article are available for a fee from The Haworth Document Delivery Service [1-800-HAWORTH, 9:00 a.m. - 5:00 p.m. (EST). E-mail address: getinfo@haworthpressinc.com].

23

I became a consumer (or client) at the mental health center in 1987 following my first psychotic break. I am here today because I was given the opportunity to start my life over again. I am here now because I believe I found my work niche, my calling.

I am a mental health provider and currently work as a Wellness and Support Advocate at Wyandot Mental Health Center (WMHC) in Kansas City, Kansas. I am also a consumer provider. (Consumer providers are persons who work in professional mental health positions but who also acknowledge and disclose their mental illness.) My job is to assist consumers in achieving levels of wellness that promote self-management of symptoms, prevent relapse, eliminate hospitalization, and assist with an individual's integration in the community. I am also involved as the executive director in our local consumer-run organization, S.I.D.E., Inc. I love the people I work with and the environment we are in together.

Consumer providers deliver the collective strength of hope and provide a positive role model for their peers. Their common experiences and familiar stories inspire and promote recovery from mental illness. Having a person beside you who has lived the life of the primary consumer and is walking the walk of recovery motivates consumers. Consumer providers are achieving goals of work, school and community integration, while at the same time managing their mental illness.

Consumer providers provide an attitude of hope for their peers–"If you can do it, maybe it's possible for me to do it, too." Consumer providers have the same work ethic as other staff. They carry the same vision and goals for their consumer peers as "professional" staff members do. However, I believe we accomplish our goals through "unique eyes and different windows of opportunity." For me, this completes the circle–it brings a healthy balance and diversity to the workplace. It can be a "win-win" situation for consumers, staff, the agency, and the entire community.

I think it is important to note, however, that getting to this place has not been an easy one for me. In fact, it has been a journey of struggles and challenges for almost twenty years. I believe most consumers do not have a goal of becoming a consumer provider. But my original career choice was to be in a helping profession. My mental illness simply gave me the direction in which to follow.

MY STORY

To know why I am here is to understand who I am and know a little bit about my story. I am a sibling in a family of ten children. Growing up, I longed to feel safe, to belong to a community, to achieve, to feel beautiful, accepted and loved. I had dreams of becoming a special education teacher, raising children and having a successful life.

My childhood experiences included a period of family trauma and abuse, but it was equally full of happy memories. We took family vacations together and shared in the adventures with all the other kids in the neighborhood. I loved to laugh, and accomplishments in school and the community came easily. I obtained a degree in special education and began working at a major medical institution as a secretary in the department of preventive medicine. I was married and busy raising three young children. I was invested in my community–its schools, churches, and neighborhoods. I valued education, justice, security, family and my spirituality. It seemed like most of my dreams were being fulfilled.

Then my world changed in a way I could never have imagined. During the summer of 1987, I experienced my first battle with an intense sadness, coupled with a lack of energy and motivation. Slowly, I could no longer keep up the pace of my work duties and the caretaking of my children. I thought this sadness was due to numerous losses I had experienced that year, including my grandmother, mother-in-law, and brother-in-law. Finally, due to the intervention of some co-workers, I found myself hospitalized for a psychiatric illness at the same medical center in which I worked. The doctors called it major depression and schizoaffective disorder. I had periods of dissociation, panic attacks, and delusions. I experienced symptoms of paranoia and anxiety, and was plagued by hallucinations. I was also confused and depressed. I simply referred to it as hell.

During this first hospitalization, I was given different colored pills to take but I didn't have a clue what they were or what they were for. I didn't like the way the side effects made me feel–stiff and lifeless. I began to unravel, feeling splintered and split apart inside. I was so scared and fearful. I was afraid of living; I was afraid of dying. I didn't feel "real." I couldn't figure out who I was or what I was becoming. The medical team told me I would get better in a year. I didn't. I found myself unable to maintain the job I had been working at for eight years. I was without a home, my marriage was failing, and I still had three children depending on me to be their mom.

My family became isolated from me. They didn't understand this illness and they weren't sure how to help. What's more, I couldn't understand it either. My perceptions of the mentally ill were of those faceless, scary, "crazy" people. Mental illness was taboo in my community–it was something that happened to the weak-minded. I couldn't under-

stand how I could be one of them. I was sure my life had been doomed to
be one of bouncing in and out of psychiatric wards, state hospitals, and
long-term care facilities. My hope for a future became dark and cloudy.

THROUGH A DIFFERENT DOOR

Because I became stuck in what seemed like the never-ending re-
volving door–in and out of the hospital–I only saw my peers when we
were very ill. The faces I saw were those of people battling the side effects of medications. They were hopeless, distraught, sad, and wander-
ing faces without names, lives or futures. This, along with my own
stereotypical conditioning and poor education, shaped my narrow focus
and allowed me to see only the label of mental illness, not the person behind it.

When I wasn't in the hospital, I attended Wyandot Mental Health
Center's day-treatment program. My case manger thought it would be a
good place for me to spend my time. It would be a place for me to get involved and it would allow me to get out of the house. It would be a place
to socialize, relax and make some new friends. I went there because I
thought it was a better option than the hospital. I thought it would be a
good place maybe to kill some time. I decided to be compliant. Besides,
I really didn't think I had much of a choice.

Being in a partial hospital program (or "day treatment" as it was
known at the time), did prove to be a good choice for me–even though I
didn't consider it so at the time. I was often restless in the highly structured program, and was bored with a regimen of "required" groups. I
didn't quite grasp how they were beneficial to me at the time. I did,
however, recognize that being in this place gave me a spark and I began
to experience tiny specks of light inside of me.

I saw faces that looked like mine. These faces reflected my own feelings and emotions. They included some of my old childhood friends,
neighbors, and church members as well as many who were unknown to
me. Some faces were of college students, parents, single moms, and
grandmothers. These faces were real, like mine. They mirrored back my
fear, confusion, anxiety, and embarrassment. They also reassured me I
wasn't alone.

With approximately 50 million Americans suffering from some form
of major mental illness (NAMI, 2000), it shouldn't have been such a
surprise to me to see these familiar faces. I ultimately came to the conclusion, which I freely share with other consumers who also have the

fear of being labeled by the mental health system, that everybody goes somewhere for something, I just happen to come here. Being part of the day program provided me the realization that there were others just like me–people I knew, and some I didn't, with their own unique story of how they came through the same door I had.

LESSONS LEARNED

This was the beginning of my awareness of what it is like to live with a mental illness. I learned that mental illness could not be all about a punishment from God. I found out that mentally ill people are not all criminals and they are not all bad, evil or possessed. I came to understand that mental illness was not my fault–that, in fact, it happens to people regardless of who they are, what they look like, or where they come from. My view of mental illness opened wide up.

I first came to the day program because I felt I had no other option. I stayed because of my peers. They provided me with friendships, safety, comfort and strength. They showed me the ropes. They pointed out the "nice" staff and they steered me away from things that needed to be avoided. These peers became my extended family, a support that was familiar to me from childhood. One woman, Gloria, became a special friend. We had grown up together and she stood by me through all my many experiences. "Cherie and I grew up together from the neighborhood," said Gloria (Personal communication, December 14, 2000). "She's like my sister. She was really scared when she came here. I pulled her up from corners. I told her to walk behind me, I would take care of her." Gloria and my peers did indeed take care of me.

I stayed involved in the day program because I knew these faces of my peers. They desired the same things I did–to feel safe and secure and to find and maintain the basic necessities that would sustain our lives. In these people, I found new friends. Friends who were people who shared many of the same dreams and goals as I did. Friends with whom I felt safe to laugh, to find moments of joy, and to be myself.

REFORM AND NEW RISK

In 1990, the Kansas Mental Health Reform Act (HB2586) became law. Words like empowerment, advocacy, and independence were suddenly on the horizon. The rally cry of the consumer movement made its way to Wyandotte County. Drop-in centers were funded through state grants. These organizations were to be designed, governed, and run by consumers. This was a brand new venture. Many of my peers were excited about this new movement. My own feelings were mixed. "This sounds good," I thought. "But can we really pull it off?"

Thanks to the wisdom and vision of our CSS Director, Leslie Young, I began to get more excited. Leslie is a person who knows a good deal when she hears one. Her outlook is always about what is best for the consumer. She gave us the push and support to develop our own drop-in center. With the support and guidance of many CSS staff, we opened our first consumer-run program. The Spectrum Drop-In Center, Inc., opened its doors for the first time in June 1992.

I was hired as one of six part-time aides. The mission of our drop-in was to provide individuals with severe and persistent mental illness a safe place to relax, socialize, build friendships, increase personal growth, awareness and self-esteem, improve social skills and enhance one's ability to live independently in the community. That was quite a challenge! My initial role as aide was to keep the center running as smoothly and efficiently as possible. This included opening and closing the center, coordinating program activities, along with some light housekeeping and clerical duties, such as answering the phones and maintaining daily attendance records and logs.

I was also hired in a separate position as a peer counselor. My role here was to support consumers who were having a hard time with the loneliness in their lives or who may be having difficulty coping with the stress of daily living. These were the informal things my peers did for me when I first came to the mental health center; it felt good to return what I had been given.

SPARKS, PUSHES, AND BUMPS

My consumer peers often talk about "turning points" or "awakenings" in their lives. I'm often asked what my turning point was. I can't lock myself into a particular time or moment that made such a dramatic difference in my life that I knew I was on a different path. As I have revisited my personal journey, I believe that my growth came in the form of little sparks, pushes, and bumps that moved me forward. What I do know to be true is that work, along with peer support, helped me reconnect to life.

Throughout my life, work has been very important to me. Achieving success and contributing to my community are values I hold very dear. Given the opportunity to work, to share my skills, education and knowledge–all things I once felt were stolen by my mental illness–gave me the needed boost and self-determination to know my life could be better. I realized that this illness didn't have to be the major controlling factor in my life. My job in Spectrum refocused my "stinky thinking." I began to dwell not on my "pity poor me" attitude but instead looked forward to new responsibilities and expectations beyond my illness. It felt good knowing that someone was counting on me to be there in the morning, to welcome and greet my friends each day. Knowing I was needed and being responsible for the operation of the center made a difference in me.

I felt empowered to make decisions that affected others and myself. My self-worth increased. My young children also reaped the benefits. They talked with their friends about what their mommy did at work. I could feel good about passing on my work values to them.

The exciting parts of being able to work started to outweigh my fears as I became used to the routine and more confident in my abilities. I realized my new responsibilities were having an impact on the way I felt about myself as a person. The label of mental illness began to diminish as I saw myself more frequently in my roles as mother, co-worker, friend, educator, advocate, and community member. I became a more integrated, whole woman with a list of strengths, not just a consumer who could *only* reach out through the eyes of an illness. I have not needed hospitalization since I began working in Spectrum fourteen years ago. That's quite a change from the average of ten per year I needed prior to this time.

I continued to work in Spectrum until 1994, having worked as the supervisor for about two years. I went to work as a VISTA volunteer for one year. I worked with a team of individuals assisting flood victims in our county with community resources. I helped clients find housing and replace household items. I also provided crisis intervention and counseling. Coincidentally, this position was located at our mental health center.

I felt nervous to be out of the safe environment of Spectrum, but I knew I could always go down the hallway for support. By working on the flood project and struggling with personnel and management issues, I was amazed at my own abilities to cope and handle tough, stressful situations. Ironically, I also observed a co-worker have the same concerns and stresses as I did, only we handled them very differently. I realized that maybe I wasn't so different from others after all.

After a year of service as a VISTA volunteer, I returned to work in the Spectrum Center. That year, our consumer board of directors faced several major challenges. They tried to keep the board together, but it soon faltered. Because the drop-in center held close ties with our mental health center (Spectrum was also housed within their building), our independent status was challenged by the state and we were denied funding for the upcoming fiscal year. Fortunately, the mental health center agreed to provide support, both financial and in-kind, and Spectrum remained open.

CONSUMER PROVIDERS MAKE A DIFFERENCE

During this transition, the one thing that remained constant was the work of the consumers who ran Spectrum. Their accomplishments and achievements were certainly noteworthy. The aides were seen as leaders and role models among their peers. They were asked by case managers to support their clients.

I felt empowered. I realized I was actually beginning to make an impact at my job. I needed less support to reach out to consumers and I was better able to see what needed to be done without a lot of structured supervision. I noticed how naturally I was able to talk to consumers. Giving support, providing encouragement, assisting with networking and working as a team to gather community resources became my priority as we worked to overcome obstacles and reach toward accomplishing personal goals. My consumer co-workers were hired as case managers, van drivers, and attendant care workers. New horizons once seen as impossible for those with the label of mental illness were becoming visible. It was exciting to be a part of history in the making.

A NEW STEP

By 1996, Spectrum had evolved to the point where it was included in the mental health center's psychosocial program. I was hired as one of two full-time aides to oversee the daily operation of Spectrum. The job was different in design than what we had experienced earlier. I was hired in a competitive position and was now considered a full-time staff. This meant I was no longer seen as a primary consumer of services at Wyandot Mental Health Center. Because of our existing policies, I could no longer come to the center for services. I experienced a loss of case management, medication clinic, and vocational services.

Even Spectrum, my most prized support base, was now my full-time place of employment. Being hired shifted the way I would receive services. I had to make the choice of receiving free services from Johnson County Mental Health Center, a center in a neighboring county, or accessing my new private health insurance. Feeling a bit rejected from the place in which I had thrived, I chose for a while to do neither.

CHALLENGES

The challenge of becoming someone who provided services to others with a mental illness was met by the fact that I was still Cherie; between the Friday I was hired and the Monday I began to work, I had not changed. I still had my illness and all the things that go along with it that make me a unique person. I remember sitting in my first "official" staff meeting and just thinking, "This is so weird, doesn't anyone else think this is strange?" I wished somebody would say something about how all this felt.

These strange feelings were accompanied by many changes. I was now a co-worker with those I had valued as *my* rehabilitation counselors, *my* vocational worker, and *my* case manager. I had so many questions. Where do I fit in with current policies, procedures and ethics? Can I talk with my co-workers about my illness? How would this affect the services of my husband who was also a consumer at our agency?

My friends and peers were now my clients. Could I still do the same things with my peers? Could we hang out? After all, we were friends and these were the people I spent my leisure time with. They had my phone number. Did I have to tell them not to call?

With the multiple roles in which I find myself involved (family member, community participant, consumer, or worker), transitioning from one role to another has sometimes been very clear and smooth. Other times it has been a major undertaking. Being a mother, wife, or church member is very clear-cut and distinct for me. My role as a consumer, however, includes many gray areas. These roles are often blurred, going from consumer to consumer-provider to staff member. There are some areas that I have found to be particularly challenging.

Initially, while working with my non-consumer co-workers, I had a feeling of being less or not equal to them. I felt I had to prove it had not been a mistake to hire me full-time. I wanted my co-workers and supervisor to see that I could do the job, and I wanted to do it perfectly. I found myself coming in earlier, along with other consumer providers, and staying later. I would volunteer to do extra outings and projects to the point of denying much needed rest and personal time for myself. Even though I have a strong work ethic, I set such unrealistic expectations of myself, expectations which were probably impossible for anyone to be successful at. However, when I didn't reach my goals, the guilt I experienced was equally high.

Another challenge revolved around confidentiality and the ethical issues regarding consumer provider roles. When I am involved in a conversation with a peer, topics may arise that require further intervention (e.g., the consumer decides to quit taking or alters his/her medication). I must decide if sharing confidential information with staff will violate the consumer's rights.

Sometimes it's a very hard job being a consumer provider, especially in situations where you have to be the "bad guy" with the people you consider your friends. I find it particularly difficult to do mediation or confront someone regarding a program violation. I have to constantly ask myself, "Is this a conflict of interest? Is this in the best interest of the consumer I'm serving?" Sometimes it feels like I have betrayed my friends and have turned into one of "them" (a non-consumer provider).

When symptoms occur while working, it can be very hard. My consumer provider colleagues and I talk about this a great deal. Despite our best efforts, we do relapse. When this happens at work, we can't just walk down the hall to see a clinic nurse or crisis case manager because of current treatment policies. It becomes a challenge for everybody involved–supervisor, team members, and the individual themselves. Relapse presents difficult and unique obstacles to intervention. Disclosure and signed releases of information help. Always we question how we will save face and return to the job after a relapse.

Taking risks and knowing my limitations are a recurring challenge. I may be unwilling to speak up for myself for fear of making waves or pointing out obvious problems ("Is what I'm feeling normal or is it related to my illness?"). Sometimes, I find myself overextending, reluctant to take annual leave days, or "stockpiling days and deeds" to ease my guilt when I do need time off.

My job in Spectrum is to give guidance and support, and to assist with mediation and conflict resolution. When I find myself in the position of having to confront my peers, it can prove to be a heart-wrenching challenge. My goal is to mediate the conflict, but I also have to work hard to maintain the relationships that I value.

Yet another challenge is knowing when and why to ask for reasonable job accommodations, which can be provided through the Americans with Disabilities Act. It is very hard for me to ask for an accommodation because I don't want my co-workers to think that I'm getting something special. I want to feel as though I am on equal ground with everyone else, even though there have been times when an accommodation would have been quite helpful.

Finally, acknowledging where I am is hard. Celebrating my strengths and accomplishments sometimes presents a fear that I will no longer be able to achieve or live up to those accomplishments. I think this comes from remembering the times when I wasn't doing as well, when I would be triggered by thoughts like, "If I am in that place again, will I be able to get out?" During these times, I can slip backward but, with the help of my co-workers and other supports, I am able to regroup and get back on track.

DISCOVERIES

I sometimes feel that I'm not quite a consumer and I'm not quite a staff member. Initially, I was trying to fit in to a place where no roads had been paved. My fellow consumer provider colleagues and I have been pioneers. We have handled each obstacle and situation as it has presented itself, and I think we have been very effective as staff.

With all the challenges facing consumer providers, one might ask why I took the risk to work in this position. Do the benefits outweigh the challenges? For me, I believe they have. I am a stronger person now and I believe that I have had an impact on the lives of my peers and within the agency. I feel proud when I see more and more of my peers stepping forward to accept the role of consumer provider. I recognize that it has been a difficult experience, but I also know the immense self-satisfaction I feel from doing a job well.

Learning, developing, exploring and growing are all processes. At our agency, we began early on to have open and honest discussions about the role of consumer providers and the impact it had on us individually and collectively, as well as on the consumer. Our agency leadership supported these early discussions and this has played a major role in the success we have had as an agency. We held forums to address expectations, concerns and attitudes on hiring consumer providers, both with staff and consumers. Though we were not always all on the same page with our feelings, the open sense of communication and forgiveness was key in my healing and in making my own role comfortable.

While it is true that all the consumer providers have not found this job to be their "niche," likewise, the hiring of "regular" staff does not always work out either. I think we have been successful because we have continued to talk about the issues. My agency did not make a big deal out of hiring consumer providers. They just did it. They stepped out of the rigid box of professional boundaries and took a risk. One of my co-workers expresses this as she talks about the growth we have experienced.

> I think we've been successful because we have continued to talk about issues as they have come up. We haven't tried to skirt around the problems or brush them under the carpet. We've been given the freedom to explore and create new things. We have created a reciprocal trust where the consumer providers have learned from the agency and the agency has learned just as much from the consumer providers. The journey of hiring consumer providers is one I would embark on again in a heartbeat. (Lori Davidson, personal communication, January 30, 2001)

The transition to providing mental health services when I was used to receiving them was indeed frightening. However, it held a deeper key to my wellness and to the wellness of my peer providers.

> When I was first hired, I wasn't really sure that I could handle the job, being that I had not worked in five years. My fears were that I would lose my medical card and social security and my only source of financial aid would be gone. I thought to myself, "What happens if I mess up? I'll get fired." So I turned to my supporters, the people who had more faith in me than I had in myself. I decided to give it a try. I did everything I could to learn my job and often worked extra because I wanted to do a good job. (Denise Baynham, personal communication, December 17, 2000)

Most of us would acknowledge that it is a good thing to be supported by others who share similar life experiences. As one who identifies as a primary consumer, I understand the devastating effects that mental illness can heap on one's life. As one who receives services, I know the contributions and talents of mental health professionals are needed and valued. I truly believe I must have an angel on my shoulder because I have been blessed throughout my services to be surrounded by support-ive, compassionate, and dedicated people.

When I first came into mental health services, the professionals rep-resented people who had all the answers; I thought they were flawless. I felt their job was to take care of me. I put them all on pedestals. I rarely saw their human side, their problems, challenges, or even their celebra-tions. They were a mystery to me. I saw each of us only in terms of one role–the "helper" and the "helpless." I also never imagined that I, too, could one day be working in this field. For me, this is the main barrier that consumer providers have broken. One of my team members ex-plains this best.

> Consumer providers have shown me the way. We've worked side-by-side for at least six years. They are my friends. These rela-tionships have inspired me to often challenge myself. I have learned that clients can see through the "professional mystique" some clinicians hold on to as if there is some secret that can't be known by all. The term "consumer provider" is a label that really only describes those individuals who have chosen to disclose their illness, but who are professionally equipped to work in the mental health field. It is, of course, paving the way for others. Perhaps this term will become more irrelevant as more individuals are recog-nized for their skill, knowledge, and unique support that they as consumer providers offer. (Personal communication, Tonya Hinman, January 14, 2001)

Consumer providers are people just like the people they serve. Many of our peers know our stories, they know the obstacles we have over-come and the challenges we face daily. Consumers can see tangible evi-dence of their peer providers working while also managing their ill-ness–taking medications, going to medicine clinics, working with their case managers, getting involved in recovery education and advocating for themselves.

Consumers witness their consumer provider peers, whom they have known or even been hospitalized with, doing positive things with their lives. I call this *believable* hope. Consumer providers are a rich source of this type of hope. Not many people like the feeling of being left out of the loop; so it is with those being served by their peers. They want to know how their consumer provider got there and what they need to do to get beyond where they are. It becomes contagious. Consumer providers serve as the motivators, the cheerleaders, and the role models while, at the same time, are known as friends.

Consumer providers are also seen as "safe" people with whom one can talk about the "hard stuff." I believe there is a higher level of trust and more open and honest communication between a consumer and a consumer provider than with professional staff. Many consumers are more at ease in discussing mental–and physical–health symptoms, medications, and side effects. It's also easier to talk with consumer providers about conflicts, daily living stresses and coping skills. Topics that may be considered taboo to talk with a staff about, like spirituality or sexuality, are generally more easily discussed with consumer providers.

Other benefits include a greater awareness of the needs of their peers. Consumer providers often demonstrate greater tolerance, patience and flexibility. They frequently have more success in engaging with consumers. Mutual support, the sharing of survival skills, and a straightforward manner of communication are often benefits consumers appreciate.

THE RECOVERY STORY

At the time I was first diagnosed with mental illness, I didn't know the "language" of recovery. I measured my own success in terms of the length of the time out of the hospital or other treatment facilities. Measures of success also included things like keeping custody of my children, being my own payee, living in my own place and participating in the mental health center's day program. This is what my co-workers and I have discussed as being "stable." I feel I was just maintaining.

Unlike fourteen years ago, we now use the word "recovery." Recovery for me now is about wellness, being responsible for my own life choices and accepting the natural consequences that occur with my decisions. Recovery is individualized and unique for everyone; we all have our own life journey. I believe it is a process of tiny steps, sparks, and bumps. I believe it parallels my own spiritual journey.

The impact of the recovery vision has helped me refocus my life. It has put my illness in perspective for me. I can now acknowledge my other life roles. Recovery enables me to have options and choices within these roles. It goes way beyond my mental illness. It has opened pathways for opportunities and new discoveries.

Most importantly, recovery has given me hope–again, a *believable* hope–for a future that I can design myself. Recovery has normalized life for me. It has been a catalyst for me to expand my world beyond the mental health world.

Recovery has also challenged the mental health system about how they deliver services to individuals with mental illness. My supervisor often talks about how things used to be and how she has seen the mentality of professionals change, especially with the advent of the recovery vision.

> We now know that recovery is more than just getting stable. For years, mental health professionals, including myself, have told consumers to take their medications, stay out of the hospital, be quiet, and don't cause problems. The goal was stability. But is stability enough? Is it enough to sit quietly in a boarding home, eat three meals a day, take your medicine, and sleep regular hours? No! In fact, it is boring and demeaning . . . Recovery is all about getting a life. The consumer movement has taught us that having hope for the future and developing meaning in your life are not just possible, but essential for all people. (Debra Hartman, personal conversation, December 19, 2000)

Recovery requires mental health centers to no longer be just programs where consumers come and participate in groups held at the center. It requires them to develop community-based services, where goals and projects are designed and developed around the consumer and in partnership with the consumer. This is the vision of community integration.

At Wyandot Mental Health Center, we are now providing recovery education to consumers through a variety of classes. "Journey of Hope" is a 9-week class which focuses on recovery as a way of confronting the effects of stigma through personal empowerment and how to rebuild and further develop personal, social, environmental and spiritual connections.

The Three R's Program: Relapse, Recovery, and Rehabilitation . . . A Wellness Approach to Psychiatric Rehabilitation is a 12-week course, taught by a psychiatric nurse, with the philosophy that education and empowerment are the keys to understand and managing psychiatric disorders. Consumer, staff and family members are educated on neurobiological brain disorders and provided with the most current information regarding the nature, course and treatment of these illnesses, as well as promoting personal and family self-awareness.

W.R.A.P., the Wellness Recovery Action Plan (Copeland, 1997), is a personal plan one creates to help him/her stay well. Through this plan, a daily "to do" list is developed to monitor health and recognize uncomfortable or distressing symptoms. It also helps consumers develop a crisis plan and other personal directives should this become necessary.

SUPPORTS

Currently, there are a growing number of supports for consumer providers. Personally, I have developed a working W.R.A.P. that I have shared with targeted supporters. I co-facilitate a consumer provider support group that meets weekly at our agency. I am involved in a coping skills group, facilitated by two other consumer providers. I participate in S.I.D.E., Inc., our local consumer-run organization and I attend other support groups when I can. I have learned basic facts about my neurobiological brain disorder, and how hope, interdependence, personal responsibility, self-advocacy, self-management of triggers and symptoms, balance, and an expanded support system enhances my recovery process.

The "Consumer as Provider" (CAPS) Training Project for consumers of mental health services, which was developed by The University of Kansas, School of Social Welfare, is an excellent opportunity for persons wanting to gain helping skills in working in human services. In the CAP class, consumers learn about basic helping and communication skills, human service work using a strengths perspective, cultural diversity, mental health care, workplace culture, employment expectations, career development, reasonable accommodations and survival skills. Each student also experiences an internship during the training at a local mental health agency that is tailored to meet the needs of the student and the agency.

> Being involved in the CAP training for me means having a job in the mental health field. It better helped me understand the consumers and the medications they are on. It helped me to open new doors. It taught me how to work well with consumers. (Kathy M., personal communication, January 12, 2001)

CURRENT TRENDS

Congress declared the 1990s the "Decade of the Brain." With the publication of the first Surgeon General's Report on Mental Health to the nation, we are breaking "best kept secrets" (U.S. Department of Health and Human Services, 1999) and individuals are being encouraged to seek treatment for mental health concerns like never before. In fact, this reports highlights the following data:

a. Mental health is essential to overall health.
b. Mental disorders are real health conditions.
c. Treatments for mental health are available and effective, and there are a wide variety of treatments available.
d. Stigma continues to prevent people from understanding that mental disorders are treatable health conditions. Stigma often keeps people from becoming full members of their community, preventing them from working, socializing, or living independently. Stigma prevents the public from a willingness to pay for care and treatment, which ultimately reduces the consumers' access to services, resources, and treatment.
e. With the emergence of stronger consumer and family-run movements, the face and direction of mental health programs will continue to improve in the upcoming years.
f. Consumer-run programs, self-help groups, and more emphasis and training for consumer self-advocacy will promote positive service and policy changes.
g. The notion of recovery reflects renewed optimism about the outcomes of mental illness, including recovery achieved through an individual's own self-care efforts. Recovery also opens opportunities for persons with mental illness to participate to the full extent of their interests in the community of their choice (U.S. Department of Health and Human Services, 1999).

As I reflect more on the concept of "consumer provider," I see my own role and position changing and evolving. The State of Kansas has now created an Office of Consumer Affairs and Development. They have also established a State Consumer Advisory Board designed to partner with Social and Rehabilitation Services to deliver the message that it is now time for the consumer's voice to be heard and their representation incorporated throughout all areas of mental health.

In the past, consumers have had little or no representation on mental health committees or boards. Fortunately, this practice is changing. I am presently serving on a statewide consumer advisory committee, and I represent our consumer-run organization on the citizens' advisory council of Osawatomie State Hospital. I am also a member of the state mental health oversight committee that is working to develop performance measures for adult and children's mental health services. Our state department of mental health also provides funding for training and consultation for a statewide consumer-run network.

This message is slowly trickling down to local mental health centers. We are currently developing a consumer affairs position for our agency, pioneering the way for other mental health centers. I will soon be moving into a new position as a consumer affairs and development specialist. I am very excited about this role. It includes participation in program design, coordination and facilitation to assure consumer participation and input. I will also be providing leadership to consumers, encouraging them to participate in decision-making and planning. I will be performing random chart reviews to assure that the center's treatment of consumers is appropriate both to the needs of the individual and guided by recovery and wellness-based philosophy and practices. I will also chair a consumer advisory board and act as liaison between the board and center management. This position will also allow me to represent WMHC on a variety of state, national, and international committees and taskforces to promote consumer awareness and involvement at all levels.

WHY I AM HERE

I am a consumer provider because it's the door I came through. Sometimes being a consumer provider is a big deal; at other times, it's no big thing. I am really no different from most of my professional co-workers. It's the nature of our jobs to do whatever is in the best interest of those we serve. My personal desire is to be a team builder. I want to bridge that which separates people, and, in the process, blur the lines of that door we came through.

As I reflect on the concept of "consumer provider," I see myself changing and evolving. I am now able to define my strengths and to see myself as someone who just happens to have an illness. My dream is a vision of recovery for all consumers.

I am a consumer provider because I am a witness to the collective strength and power of people who understand what I've been through. I feel a connection and camaraderie with my consumer peers. I carry them close in my heart. I desire to understand their challenges and embrace their accomplishments with celebration. I am a consumer provider because I want to share my believable hope.

I work as a mental health provider because I am a dreamer. I believe in the dreams of my consumer peers and I have the willingness to walk with them wherever the path might lead. I believe in miracles–in the capabilities of each individual, regardless of their illness or challenge. I know people can accomplish great things when given the appropriate supports, options, and opportunities.

I believe that suicide is not an option. It scares me when I remember and it scares me when I am there again. I know what it feels like to walk a tightrope, teetering between hope and despair. I want my peers to hold on, to receive sparks, and to grow and discover life. I want others to know that if anyone who tells them they are "less than," then those are the people I wonder about most.

I believe people deserve the chance to learn about wellness and mental health and to be further responsible for their own lives. I believe in providing windows of opportunities, taking calculated risks, and exploring all avenues of one's dreams and goals. I believe in the principles of justice, respect and dignity. I believe that I am somebody to be respected and I am deserving of the best.

I am a fighter and a survivor. I believe I can be a catalyst toward eliminating stigma in my community. To see yourself in the role of being "mentally sick" sucks the desire of living right out of a person. Stigma cuts deep into the soul. As a black woman, I have encountered stigma all my life, but nothing compared to the stigma I have endured because of my mental illness. I believe it is my obligation to help educate others and help my neighbors and community know that I–and my peers–are more than just our illness.

I work because I believe in recovery. I work because I want my peers to find joy in living. I work because I want to continue to achieve, grow, and contribute. I am here today because I truly think it is my spiritual destiny and my life's journey to have a career in human services. I cannot think of a place I would rather be.

ACKNOWLEDGMENTS

I would like to thank the following people:

- My early case managers, especially Dawn and Kay, who helped bring me back.

- My vocational counselor, Lisa, who pushed me down the hall.
- Tonya and Lori, who are my mentors, my role models, and especially, my friends.
- My fellow pioneer, Denise, who is my best friend and always there.
- The many other consumer providers I have had the privilege to work with; your courageous spirit inspires me.
- My current case manager, Patricia, who's putting it all into perspective for me.
- My family–Ronnie, O.J., Cherie, and Cee Cee–my best supporters.

REFERENCES

Copeland, M.E. (1997) *Wellness recovery action plan.* W. Dummerston, VT: Peach Press.

Moller, M.D., & Murphy, M.F. (1998). *The three R's program: Relapse, recovery, and rehabilitation . . . A wellness approach to psychiatric rehabilitation.* Nine Mile Falls, WA: Author.

National Alliance for the Mentally Ill (NAMI). (2001). *Facts and figures about mental illness* [Brochure]. Arlington, VA: Author. [Available online at http://www.nami.org/fact.htm]

U. S. Department of Health and Human Services. 1999. Mental Health: A Report of the Surgeon General. Rockville, M.D.: U. S. Department of Health and Human Services, Substance Abuse and Mental Health Services Administration, Center for Mental Health Services, National Institutes of Health, National Institute of Mental Health.

Where the Rainbow Speaks
and Catches the Sun:
An Occupational Therapist
Discovers Her True Colors

Suzette (Susan) Mack, OTR

SUMMARY. Living with a neurobiological brain disorder, commonly known as a mental illness, requires a lifetime of diligent work toward recovery and wellness. This paper outlines the story of one occupational therapist's journey with her own mental illness. She prefers to call her own road of "recovery" one of "discovery," as it has led her to discover true talents and gifts (strengths) even amongst encounters with old models that emphasize weaknesses and disability over abilities and capabilities. The following journey unfolds as advances in research, changes in services, increased focus on consumer as leader and increased tools and resources available lead the way toward a more positive ability to live a purposeful life, engaging in meaningful activities in spite of an illness. This paper gives a personal account as a tool to be used by other therapists as they travel along their own treatment journeys–whether with, or as consumers, of mental health services. *[Article copies available for a fee from The Haworth Document Delivery Service: 1-800-HAWORTH. E-mail address: <getinfo@haworthpressinc.com> Website: <http://www.HaworthPress. com> © 2001 by The Haworth Press, Inc. All rights reserved.]*

Suzette (Susan) Mack is a graduate student at the University of Kansas, Lawrence.

[Haworth co-indexing entry note]: "Where the Rainbow Speaks and Catches the Sun: An Occupational Therapist Discovers Her True Colors." Mack, Suzette. Co-published simultaneously in *Occupational Therapy in Mental Health* (The Haworth Press, Inc.) Vol. 17, No. 3/4, 2001, pp. 43-58; and: *Recovery and Wellness: Models of Hope and Empowerment for People with Mental Illness* (ed: Catana Brown) The Haworth Press, Inc., 2001, pp. 43-58. Single or multiple copies of this article are available for a fee from The Haworth Document Delivery Service [1-800-HAWORTH, 9:00 a.m. - 5:00 p.m. (EST). E-mail address: getinfo@haworthpressinc.com].

KEYWORDS. Wellness recovery action plan, strengths model, dissociation, consumer provider, bipolar disorder

It's January 21st, 1963–one of the coldest days Chicago has ever had. My mom is back at the hospital and it looks like the labor pains are for real this time. I'm born–at last! The third girl, only my parents are both excited. Everything seems healthy. I have all my fingers, all my toes. My arms and legs are healthy, my vision seems fine and I am eating without much prompting. My mom can finally relax after many months of worried prayers that her baby would be healthy. (You'll have to remember that this was the era of "DES" babies; only no one knew exactly what was causing all those terrible birth defects at this time, people were just plain scared that their babies would be affected.)

It's Autumn 1963. President Kennedy has been fatally wounded, the weather is getting chilly again, and I continue to be a screaming child, who is failing to thrive. I'm back in the hospital again, with the nurses taking turns rocking me (hhhmmm, wonder if there was an OT on staff doing some intervention?!) . . . not that I'd fall asleep. I just kept on screaming. Food allergies, the doctor decided. I'm on goat's milk now and doing so much better. I've gotten this little bulging tummy and my skin isn't red anymore. But I continue to have a lot of difficulty relating calmly to my environment. It's hard for others to interact with me. I'm not always the type of child people rush over to gush over–especially when I am screaming.

I'm four now. I didn't talk until I was three and everything seems to make me nervous and fretful. I have so much excessive energy that my superstitious grandmother thinks Lucifer is in me. One afternoon, I wake up from a nap having some sort of partial seizure–the type where the brain activity in the temporal lobe goes awry. Imagine being four and feeling like your limbs are too heavy, feeling out of your body, seeing things that really aren't there. I try to tell my mom (this thing's really hard to explain, I just know I'm very scared) . . . only nobody knows what's going on, so life goes on as usual for all of them . . . only for me, nothing feels right inside my head or my body ever again. It's hard to develop normally–to laugh and play–when you never know when things will suddenly feel so funny.

I'm seven, eight, nine and ten–having a lot of problems with school phobia. It's not that I don't like school, it's just that weird things happen to me when I'm sitting under the fluorescent lights at school. These sensations also happen when I have to sit in the big gymnasium with hundreds of other students during "fun" special events–and also when I'm in the noisy cafeteria during lunch, riding the school bus and playing on the playground. Actually, I'm beginning to dread school because it makes the weird things inside my head even scarier. It's not just school where I have these things happen to me–it's in church, at the store, even at home sometimes. I begin to discover that when I am at home and go someplace quiet–and especially when I write in my diary–that my mind begins to quiet and my center place returns. I miss a lot of school, but my grades are pretty good so nobody seems to notice. I'm pretty withdrawn at school and have a hard time making friends. There's so much going on inside my body to pay attention to, that I all but miss what's going on around me.

I'm eleven and becoming a young lady! Hormones are shifting and I'm begging to get my ears pierced. My friends and I talk on the phone. A lot. I'm busy with our horses, playing my cello and helping take care of all the little foster brothers and sisters that come to live in my home. I still have weird things happen, but I've gotten more used to them. Until one night. I'm lying in bed and this major hallucination, out of body thing starts to happen. I turn over, I pray, I sing inside my head, I take deep breaths–it doesn't stop. I scream for my mom and end up in the hospital. "Anxiety" the doctor says and puts me on some sort of pill that makes me sleep on and off for three days straight. I wake up tired, afraid and embarrassed. Only no one seems to understand–actually, no one really wants to talk about it. I learn to keep it to myself and live an adolescence of inner angst that slowly leads to a major depression, marked with lots of those "weird" things happening without warning and lasting for unpredictable lengths of time. I learn to not trust doctors–they don't seem to understand anything I tell them and they seem only to talk to my parents and tell them things like "She's just stressed." I ask myself why my brother and sisters aren't so stressed . . .

I'm in high school now. My hormones are straightening out. I'm 16 and 17 and really pretty happy. I still can't tolerate fluorescent lights or noisy, stimulating places but I've learned to compensate by avoiding them as much as possible. My depression and anxiety are still there; I write poetry and journal a lot and that really seems to help. I draw in black and white pencil and charcoal too, to reflect my mood and express the inner turmoil that no one sees, but that ravages my soul with its unpredictability and viciousness. This thing is robbing so much of my childhood, but thank goodness I don't seem to realize it. There are also times when I am very happy and energetic. There's even this one time when some of my teachers call a conference with my mom and the principal to discuss what they feel must be "a problem with alcohol." (Heck, it's just undiagnosed mania, so leave me alone. I'm rather liking all this up time after having so little of it the last few years!) They let me off the hook; after all, my grades are good and no one can prove it. Two of my friends confront me, wondering if I am doing drugs. I'm not and I laugh at their perplexed faces when they tell me that if not drugs, then what is causing me to have so much energy. I misbehave in classes and get asked to leave. I think it's funny to be so hyper. I'm having so much fun and have no idea what scars my erratic behavior is having on my development. Isn't it normal adolescence to not understand consequences, to use poor judgement, to have little splits with reality where you sort of become someone you really aren't?

Halfway through my senior year a guy in one of my classes puts drugs in my food. He thinks it's going to be really funny–but instead, I get really, really ill and life will never be the same for me again. My already shaky brain chemistry takes this opportunity to shows its evil side, and things goes very awry for me for a very, very long time. The olfactory and visual hallucinations are awful. They tell me I'm having "flashbacks." I never know when it will happen, and because I don't know what it all means, I learn to be afraid–phobic is more the word. I'm scared to go out in public, scared to eat food, scared to drive and scared to be at work. I'm scared of movements, I'm scared of heights, I'm scared of so much–my life is becoming smaller and smaller. The times when I can sit home near my mom in quietness and structure are just about the only times I know I'll be okay–even if this monster rears itself inside my brain. This thing in my head has already marred my social development. Now it's making things even worse than ever before. I pray for relief, I pray that I will wake up "cured" and "back" on this earth again. It doesn't happen and I become exhausted, sadder, more anxious and less whole than ever before. I am afraid that maybe it's the food I'm eating that makes me feel so weird, so I start to eat only certain things and the onset of a brand new thing the doctors later call "anorexia nervosa" begins.

Full of paranoia and suspiciousness, markedly depressed, anxious, intermittently hallucinating, showing symptoms of dissociating–this is how I enter college in 1981. While others are enjoying meeting new friends, walking with newfound freedom around the huge Colorado campus in Boulder, and honing in on who they're going to be for the rest of their lives, I'm fighting off demons that make concentration nearly impossible. I seek relief from a doctor, who sends me to a psychiatrist. I learn biofeedback, take a bunch of tests, find out I have "temporal lobe" epilepsy, and continue to be so affected by a perpetuating neurobiological brain disorder (that's the newest term for "mental illness" . . . wish that terminology and understanding had been around before the '90s) that life is anything but normal for this college gal.

College is a struggle for me. I have to sit in the back of the classroom to avoid being overstimulated. It's hard for me to concentrate and I have episodes of depression that mark me as an outcast in comparison to my chipper colleagues who love to go to Buff's football games, drink cheer with friends and travel to sunny beaches during semester breaks. I stay in a bad relationship way too long. I'm fascinated with psychology and science and begin to break away from my journalism major into more existential searchings behind the meaning of existence and the reasons for behavior. I graduate in 1986; it took me extra long because I kept needing to take time away from my studies due to health issues. I'm working a couple of part-time jobs but struggling really hard. My psychiatric symptoms are overwhelming me, but I've learned not to talk about it any more because the labels I've gotten are anything but accepted by the mainstream medical field I'm in–and I've discovered that after the labels have been noted in my medical chart, I'm somehow treated differently–with derogatory cynicism and neglect. There's this one time when I'm really ill. I've had a horrible sore throat, fever and headache for several weeks. My usual doctor won't do any tests. They tell me it's all stress, that I need to exercise more and that I'm making things up. I end up at a different clinic where no one knows my records. I get treated like a human being and find out I have mono. Thanks doc.

It's 1988. I've had this horrible battle with depression and anorexia for the last 18 months. I'm married now, only my husband moved to work in another state and I'm not coping very well. I continue to hallucinate and dissociate. I continue to be very afraid of the symptoms I experience and have absolutely no idea what is going on. I'm certain I have demons–stress, anxiety, something I have done wrong to deserve what's going on. It's hard to concentrate on the world around me. I'm surprised I'm able to function at all–but I do, sort of. I need time away from my job to be hospitalized. I hate it there. The staff is rude–they carry in fast food and laugh over self-indulgent lunches, while making all of "us" sit in a circle in the main hospital dining room eating whatever is served to us, whether we like it or not (or whether or not we're vegetarians, Jewish, hypoglycemic or just plain people with food preferences like everybody else). They make us do these affirmations before and after we eat. That's greatly humiliating when all the "normal" people at the tables around us stop to watch and whisper. Under the fluorescent lights I fail to thrive even less than I was when I entered that place. They put me on the medical floor and my depression and shame spiral even further downward. One of the nurses who treats me knows me from before I was so ill–she wants to know what's gone so wrong in my life. I shut my eyes and close the blinds. I pretend not to hear her in the hall talking about how scared she is that my resting pulse is only 40 and that my kidneys don't seem to be working very well right now.

I let myself out of that place. My doctors don't agree with my decision. I go to my parents house for awhile. I am pretty sick. I am very weak. I am skinny and malnourished, depressed and alone. I've learned that when I undereat the junk in my head quiets down. I get this runner's high sort of feeling that lasts until my blood sugar crashes so badly I can barely see. My body hurts. I bruise easily. I wear three sweaters when others wear only tee shirts. It ruins my immune system and ruins my career. It ruins my marriage and it ruins my self-esteem. But at least for awhile the demons are gone and there is peace inside when for so long there's only been war. I'm running on empty emotionally, spiritually and physically but I keep on finding the reasons for the lessons life is giving me. I'm determined to stay strong, determined to fight the battles that lie ahead. I don't realize how much my reality is askew by all of this. I don't realize that it isn't normal to be depressed, to dissociate, to not have goals to reach toward. I don't realize it isn't normal to be so reactive to the world around me. I don't realize I'm having internal hallucinations. I just know something is wrong and that no matter how hard I fight to feel normal again, nothing seems to work.

I want to know what's wrong with me. I start to study books in the library about neurology. I enroll in anatomy and physiology at the junior college nearby. I have a friend drive me to and from classes, and sit with me while I study. I have trouble doing things alone because of my illness. I'm having episodes of agoraphobia again, and of course, I'm still very anorexic. But I'm starting to become so enthralled with the human body that nothing matters anymore except making sure I understand every little detail my professors are relaying. During times when the pain is too much, I'm learning how to put myself into altered states where I see bright white lights and angels. It's very reassuring, no matter how weird this sounds. I can feel the angels' wings protecting me. I don't have any clue how different other people's lives my age are and how I'm missing out on most of my 20's. I can't remember if anyone's mentioned medications except for anxiety reducers–which carry labels and stigmas and almost-certain addiction. People just keep telling me to eat and that if I'd be more self-empowered I'd never have gotten into this predicament to start with. This only makes me isolate more, withdrawing into a rather unsafe place. Don't you think if there was something I could do to change my world, that I'd be doing it?

I explore careers a little bit more. I get accepted to a physician assistant program but turn it down. I know I'm too "ill" to go. I get accepted to a top-notch nursing program. A nurse friend of mine talks me out of it and tells me about her favorite people to work with–occupational therapists. I explore this career and shadow some therapists at the hospitals in my city. I am intrigued by this profession and begin to take the prerequisites for the program at Colorado State University. I do it all–in spite of the fact that my body weight is dangerously low, that my depression invades my very essence and that I have become so ashamed of myself that the only thing I have to turn to is my studies. It's the only time I know that I have something to contribute. I'm on a journey to self-discovery–a journey to define what many of the professionals I've seen have marked with the scarlet labeling of insanity. I'm also on a journey to help others who struggle in similar battles and to do something positive with the struggles I experience. I have episodes when I need to be hospitalized during this time. I am blessed with a boss who is flexible and lets me do some of my work from home. Two of my doctors try to convince the others that I am unable to make decisions for myself. I have one who befriends me and that is all that I need to boost my morale up to the place it needs to be when I officially enter my studies in occupational therapy at Colorado State University in 1995.

I know deep inside, before I even know that much about occupational therapy, that this is the career that fills in the gaps that other health care professionals leave out. This is the field that looks at what happens at school, at home, at work and at play, when someone is sick–or somehow different than what would be expected by "the norm." This is the field that examines the body as an integrated self. This is the field that uses theory, biology, common sense and a whole lot of humanity to treat the person as abled, not disabled–as whole, not broken–and a field that isn't afraid to join the hands of the people it works with in an attempt to a build a partnership, instead of a perpetuating barricade.

It's 1995. I'm very ill. My eating disorder is taking over my being. My depression makes my thoughts miserable–and that's on my good days. My immune system is really suppressed and it's causing cognitive problems, such as memory holes and confusion. I'm given the diagnoses of chronic fatigue syndrome and fibromyalgia. I know that I am ill and immediately get a whole team of health professionals involved with my care when I move to Fort Collins to start school. I have a dietician, an internist, a psychotherapist and a neurologist. I find a minister to be guided along in my spiritual journey. I begin to make a few friends and I confide in a professor some things about my illness. I start learning about the newly enforced Americans with Disabilities Act. I request accommodations for my illness, only focusing on the eating disorder's effects on my physical health. I'm told I have mono again. I need a handicapped parking sticker because I am too weak to walk around campus to my classes. I spend a lot of time alone and have difficulty with roommates. I avoid a lot of social situations–especially if they deal with food. I refuse to tell any of my classmates about my illness. I begin to feel like a failure as I notice my energy level being so different than everyone else's. I am very, very ashamed. I am confronted, nicely, by one of my peers about being so thin. She becomes an advocate, having recovered from an eating disorder herself. I feel encouraged and work very hard at school. My grades are good, my courage is strong, but my health continues to suffer. I wake up sometimes in the middle of the night and realize I am completely trapped by this thing, no matter how hard I try to overcome it, or how much treatment I receive. I just don't seem to be pulling out of all of this very quickly, that's for certain.

It takes me an extra year to finish school. I graduate with a group of people I hardly know and end up in two classes' "graduating" picture. My ability to rebound is tapering and sometimes I feel like I'm losing grounds with my mental illness. I know I am sick, but am too full of guilt, embarrassment and shame to reach out in any real way. I'm tired of seeing people point at me and whisper. "Yes, I'm thin–so what!?" I want to scream, but can't find my voice when I want to yell. I'm going through a divorce. I'm losing my will to live. My doctors recommend lithium. Then they recommend valium. One tells me to exercise, the other one tells me to rest. They recommend this, then that . . . during my psychosocial OT class my professor makes a big deal out of eating disorders and I hear two of my classmates making fun of hallucinations. I'm tired of it all. I'm tired of not being able to reach out in trust to anyone. I'm tired of not being courageous enough to stand up for the rights of those with mental illnesses–I'm too unempowered to know that it's not something we have caused ourselves, but something that is neurobiologically wrong within our bodies. I am tired of trying to "solve myself." I just want to be left alone. I start regretting my studies in OT. I feel confused about everything right now and really don't trust my teachers. It may sound angry or unfeeling, but I don't find a lot of my peers to be particularly understanding about what it really means to have issues that require occupational therapy. I feel like "patients" are looked at as "projects to dissect." I like it when we start calling them clients and learn about "watching our language." I know good things are coming in the arena of healthcare when it concerns treating people as respectable human beings. I am in a city where holistic and alternative healthcare is readily explored and I start learning about massage, meditation, aromatherapy, Eastern medicine, Native American spirituality and a lot of other non-medical model approaches to wellness and wholeness–and I know that's the way I want to practice therapy.

I start applying the things I'm learning as an OT student to myself. I write down what is purposeful activity for my own life, sort out my life domains, and start working hard at doing "normal" things for me to see if that will help my illness abate. I start to take tap and modern dance lessons and spend a lot of time tending to herbs in a friend's garden. I start to write again and get hired to write a medical column for the campus newspaper. I start taking ballet and ballroom dancing lessons and learn that doing the turns is helping integrate my nervous system. I feel stronger, more assertive and less ashamed. I am working very conscientiously at being strong and not having the symptoms of my illness domineer my life, although admittedly I am still not really sure what my illness is all about.

I face Level II internships. I need special accommodations and get special priority so I can do mine locally. The stress of relocating would be too difficult on my health. I continue to struggle with peers who have negative attitudes toward me–thinking I am slacking when it's not about that at all. I silently cry, wondering why they just don't seem to "get" how sick I am and how much I covet their strong legs and healthy brains that let them ride fantastic journeys I'll never be able to touch. It's hard to know what is real anymore when I start my first internship at a long term care facility. The physical disability part of this internship is difficult for me as I work hard to apply the theory I've learned in the classroom setting–but it's funny how almost instinctually I understand the psychological and neurological needs of a lot of the clients that my supervisor and I treat. I go on to my second internship and work with in an out-patient brain injury recovery program. Again, I find myself relating deeply to the emotional impact of the transitional and role-changing issues these clients are going through. More than this, I'm beginning to find out more about antidepressant medications, hallucinations and seizures. These are things that I've had some encounters with–but never before have they been so real. It's hard to give my full attention to my clients when I am in need of so much care myself, but I give it my best effort and work very hard to complete my credentials. I don't want anyone to know how sick I feel, nor what bad thoughts keep going through my head all the time–thoughts that make no matter what I'm doing the wrong thing; thoughts that question every move I make, make me feel inadequate and make my mind race so badly I never wake up feeling refreshed.

It's January 1995. I'm driving to Denver to take the national certification exam for occupational therapists. I'm still not feeling all that well and have had a couple of emergency room visits lately. There's other stuff going on with my health, but I figure it's all about my eating disorder. I don't realize the other stuff that's going on–like how I dissociate and how much being depressed has impaired my ability to relate with others, clouded my life, dreams and hopes and how much it is going to impact my future. As I sit and take the exam, I get this sense that I am not really certain I'll be a good clinical occupational therapist. I believe I'd be much better doing some sort of research, but I also know I need a few good years in the field as a practitioner to lend credibility to anything else I may aspire to in this profession. I concentrate hard and three months later am celebrating with my peers the passing of our exams!

It's March 1995 now. I interview for a job in Kansas doing long term care. I am a little scared of being so far from home but am determined not to be ill anymore. One week after my interview I find out I have cancer. You know, when life hits you hard, sometimes it just isn't ready for the bruises to heal. Anorexia is hard to hide. Everyone can see it when they look at you. But you don't have to tell anyone if you don't want to. You can say no to treatment, no to medication, and certainly no to food. You can hide, in full confidence that you're pretty much in control. You know your body better than most doctors with 25 years of experience. You're on your way to getting your unofficial degrees in nutrition and physiology. Your electrolytes get off, you faint a couple of times and your heart skips around a bit–so you call your doctor or drink a sports drink, and life returns to its restricted, puny self in spite of your illness. But with cancer it's different. I was so upset that I told my doctor "no way" to his treatment demands, got in my car, and headed toward the ocean. I stopped and turned around. I knew I couldn't run and hide from this one. My doctor pleaded for me to listen–he told me he wouldn't let this be my way out, that there was treatment, that he believed I'd make the right choice, that my eating disorder had nothing to do with this cancer so I could quit feeling so guilty. I was in the emergency room one night and my doctor wasn't there. One of his colleagues was on duty and shared with me his personal experience with cancer, and pleaded with me to listen. I listened and I understood. I had hope again and partook in their meal toward wellness. But I also knew that even though the cancer was "gone" according to my doctor, holistically I had a lot of healing left to do. He didn't like it when I told him so–just blamed it all on my depression.

In July 1995 I move to Kansas to begin working in long term care facilities. I was scared, uncertain, but excited and hopeful. I wanted to be a good representative of the occupational therapy profession. I was determined to do the best that I could. I was still undereating, still horribly depressed–but took a personal vow to be in recovery (as if I could do that all by willpower). I'm learning a lot and focusing hard on being the best occupational therapist I can be for all the people I worked with and among. I take my job very seriously and make it a priority to treat the people as "people first." I think it is because I have been through so much myself that my level of compassion is so high. I work hard to educate other staff members about the transitional issues the elderly are facing when they are uprooted from their homes, taken from spouses and lose their independence and health to move into a skilled nursing facility. I teach others about purposeful activity and work hard with the activity departments to find ways to keep residents away from chronic sitting in wheelchairs all day long, doing nothing except waiting for the next meal, bedtime and slipping away into sad thoughts and meaningless, hopeless days. I do my own informal review of residents' charts and wonder why at least 75% of them are on an antidepressant . . .

Things go fairly well for about a year. I'm still having trouble with depression, but am finding new friends and things to do that break up the lonely times I spend alone after work. I don't know when it started, but the racing thoughts are back. They make me never rest in anything I do–I have to keep on pushing ahead, trying to find happiness, meaning and purpose in life. I take dance classes, enroll at several classes at the local university, get overly busy with my church and various volunteer activities. I get ritualistic about eating and won't allow myself to eat unless I've pushed really hard all day long. My thoughts are obsessive, my mind races–and I never really feel happy. Just sad, alone and weary from a mind that won't shut up. I find out I have a problem with an overactive thyroid. This explains some of that racing stuff. I start dating a guy in 1997. My eating disorder kicks in again–and I don't have much reserve for this to happen.

It's June of 1998. I'm practicing some dancing for a workshop I'm going to lead at my church. The custodian is there and washes the floor in the area I'm jumping and leaping around. He forgets to put up signs to warn of wet floors and I have a slip and fall accident. I hit the back of my head really hard and injure the occipital lobe. It takes a while to heal but I'm left with some visual disturbances, including visual hallucinations. I now know what it means to have some delayed symptoms from a head injury. I keep trying to do clinical work in occupational therapy but it's getting harder because of all the symptoms I am having with my mental illness, and now the head injury on top of it. Really, I am not a malingerer, nor am I in hypochondriasis. This stuff is really happening no matter how "well" I am trying to be. I don't know it now, but I will be learning soon that part of wellness means knowing how to live with a chronic thing like mental illness, and not trying to never have symptoms or think you can overcome them entirely. It's as chronic, and needs as much daily attention, as something like diabetes.

It's January 1998. I am in a fog. I can no longer cope with my daily life and work because of my illness. I am in the middle of a break from reality. This is very hard to talk about . . . and extremely hard to endure. I am in a town where people, including physicians, don't understand that mental illness is as much neurophysiological as it is behavioral. I am ridiculed and treated less than human. I escape by moving to Kansas City where I do receive better health care, support and begin a whole new adventure in learning about mental illness–and personal recovery.

I'm told I am bipolar and that is why I am having the ups and downs. I begin receiving services at Wyandot Mental Health Center in Kansas City–case management, psychiatry and counseling. I am isolated for awhile from everyone there except my direct treatment providers. It's safer this way and I don't think I have much in common with the other consumers there. Looking back I know I am totally ashamed of my illness and the nervous collapse I had. I didn't do justice to the occupational therapy world. I let my family, friends and future down and felt deep shame for this. I do a lot of soul searching and praying and decide not to practice clinically for awhile. I have to get my symptoms managed.

I refuse hospitalization even though every one of my providers is encouraging it. My significant other also wants me to go to the hospital. I just keep on trying hard to find purpose in life and engage in meaningful activities. I think that will solve all my problems. I take classes at a community college and try out my writing skills for a local health newspaper. I don't believe the hospital will help–I believe I will be over medicated and not listened to. I believe that staff will treat me with disdain and punish me for having an illness that displays itself so emotionally and behaviorally. I don't know this at the time but some of my trust issues are due to the paranoia that comes along with my illness.

I just want to be "better" and "gainfully" employed again, yet I have no idea of who I am or what I will do with my life now that I am not practicing occupational therapy. This is a rough road to be on. I know there are many paths along the journey in life, but part of the problem with my brain makes me see and consider all the options at once. I am so overwhelmed with them that it is impossible to make choices, to concentrate or to hold down even entry level jobs. I try a variety of medications. I have side effects that scare me. I quit the meds and keep on trying it alone, not realizing how typical this pattern is among people with severe mental illnesses.

It's January of 1999. I find out about a pilot program being offered through the University of Kansas' School of Social Welfare. It's called "Consumers As Providers" (CAPS). It is a 20-week commitment to classes and fieldwork designed to enable people who use mental health services find employment within mental health centers. There are 12 students in the class. Our educational levels range from non-high school graduate to doctorate level graduate. Some of us have never been able to work; others have been professionals who have been forced out of their realm due to illness. All of us want a chance to find employment and purpose in life. All of us work hard to discover our true talents and what it will mean to work with accommodations. We work under Charles Rapp's "Strengths Model," which sees a person's strengths, not weaknesses and gives hope where gloom may once have stolen happy thoughts and forward motion. I see a lot of similarities in Rapp's work to occupational therapy theories, and find it comforting to be part of a program that sees the person and ability first over any "disability."

It's a good experience. I do my fieldwork at Wyandot Mental Health Center in their "Wellness" department and get hired in June of 1999 as a part-time advocate. I am not directly practicing occupational therapy there, but work among OT students and apply my knowledge and skills as an OT in the work I do with adults who have severe and persistent mental illnesses.

I am one of several mental health consumers hired as employees to bring special insights and experiences that non-consumer employees cannot. We all learn first hand how hard it is to become an employee at a place you once received services (or still receive). There are many boundary issues and part of my job is to work the "Strengths Model" and to break down the "us and them" boundaries that threaten to put a barrier between "staff" and "consumers." To see us as capable instead of incapable . . . to trust us and treat us as equals . . . to give us a chance when we've only received discouragement . . . these are a few of our goals. Being a "Consumer Provider" presents many unexpected issues. Once I told my case manager I was struggling with stress on my job. She, in good faith, told my supervisor without my permission, thus breaking confidentiality rules. After many meetings and much contemplation, new policies were put into place regarding similar situations. Another difficulty is being in meetings as an employee where my providers were present. Talk about role confusion! Another thing I struggle with is feeling underemployed and not as challenged as I had as an O.T. I had accommodations that enabled me to work, but felt my employer's expectations of my work were lower than for non-consumer employees.

Working at Wyandot Mental Health Center provided me the opportunity to receive ongoing education. These workshops, classes and inservices served a dual purpose for me–education to apply to myself, as well as to the consumers I worked among. One particularly interesting and helpful 12-week course is entitled "The 3 R's," which stand for recovery, relapse and rehabilitation. Created by a nurse (Mary Moller), this course details the major mental illnesses (bipolar disorder, depression, schizophrenia), teaching what they are, how to treat them and ways to prevent relapse. As we studied parts of the brain and discussed lifestyle adaptations to promote wellness, I felt as if I were back in occupational therapy school again. Another helpful recovery tool I use is based on Mary Ellen Copeland's work. Entitled "WRAP" (which stands for Wellness Recovery Action Plan), this empowering concept teaches consumers to design personal plans to maintain wellness, recognize triggers and symptoms, and to implement a pre-planned protocol when times get rough. This is an excellent tool that virtually anyone might benefit from, since we all experience highs and lows in life.

I learn a lot but find I need to quit my job in March of 2000 because I am getting ill again. I find a job working as an editor for a Website. When I am working alone and focusing on writing, the severity of my symptoms are so much less. It is a nice retreat from the chaos that goes on within my brain. I am seriously depressed and have a lot of confusion about who I am and what to do next with my life. I know I need to be on medications, yet I keep fighting it. I'm running out of reserves though and headed for trouble.

It's August of 2000. I am really on the downward part of my spiral. I end up in the hospital for one week because of suicidal depression and weight loss that is causing heart irregularities. I then go to an eating disorders program for about two months. I am diagnosed with Graves' disease (hyperthyroidism) and told that it is contributing to my rapid weight loss, shakiness, weakness, racing thoughts and symptoms of psychosis. I start taking an antidepressant, mood stabilizer, antiseizure medication and antipsychotic. I also receive treatment for Graves' disease, which can create symptoms of psychosis. I spent all day in a variety of groups learning coping skills for the eating disorder. I get back in touch with my higher power. I am learning more about wellness now and beginning to see a light again in my life instead of gloominess and darkness. The suicidal feelings abate. I feel like engaging in life again. I am scared to leave the hospital, but know that at some point wellness for me must take place outside the sheltered walls of an institution, even though there is still progress to be made when it comes to the treatment of the mentally ill. I have learned to use meditation, dance, exercise, journaling, drawing, deep breathing and a myriad of artistic expressions of self as ways to help maintain wellness. I've learned to reach out to others, to rely on their strength when mine is wavering. My shame is a lot less now and a spirit of acceptance surrounds my soul. I feel prepared again to contribute to the field of occupational therapy, especially in the psychosocial arena.

I was asked to contribute to this publication to discuss my illness and talk about recovery. To me, recovery is a life-long process . . . not so much one of regaining or "atoning," but a journey of discovering one's true colors and letting them shine on through in spite of the fog that sometimes clouds the rainbow. Those who know me well know that I prefer the term "discovery" to "recovery," for I find it less shaming and blaming and more hopeful and enriching. I now feel that I am healthy in spite of my illness, in spite of my diagnosis and in spite of all the tough times I have had in my life. I know I face a lifetime of medications. I know I face a lifetime of learning to live in a state of empowerment and wellness in spite of this neurobiochemical imbalance. There are still so many ways occupational therapists can contribute to the world of mental illness. I have had the privilege of being part of the CAPS program and subsequently working for a year within a very progressive community mental health setting. I have had the privilege of returning to work in a very sheltered environment, one in which I could openly share the details about my illness and receive accommodations without having to fear repercussions. I was also part of creating a drama/dance troupe in which its performers tell their stories of what it is like to have a mental illness to a variety of groups as a way to educate and advocate for their community. The troupe is called "True Colors" and does a beautiful dance to Cyndi Lauper's song by the same name. It is available to perform for those interested.

When I am asked if I am well, I now say "yes." When asked if I have side effects from my medications, the answer is the same. If asked if I will ever practice occupational therapy clinically again, the answer is "yes"–but my inner spirit tells me my work will never be the same again. My personal road of discovery is not over, as I am pursuing continued education in the field of nursing, where I feel my talents will be best used. I hope that my story provides hope and insight. If it lends courage to but one person, then I have done my job. I also offer myself to anyone who might want to tell his or her own story, or might wish for me to elaborate on any part of mine to further empower and better the treatment of the mentally ill. One last comment I'd like to make is this: if it seems as if I have had a myriad of diagnoses, this is partially true. As we experience medical advances, research, diagnostics and treatment will also be enhanced. As all astute occupational therapists know, we have to peel away what we see one layer at a time–the proverbial "activity analysis" in full action . . . and to make a commitment to seeing the strengths of all whom we are privileged to work among. Remember, it is among the full spectrum of colors in which we see the true radiance of the rainbow of life.

REFERENCES

1. Lauper, Cyndi. "True Colors."
2. Mary Ellen Copeland, MS, MA. Wellness Recovery Action Plan. 1997. Peach Press, United States.
3. Mary Moller, MSN,ARNP, CS and Millene Freeman Murphy, Ph.D, APRN, CS. Recovering from Psychosis: A Wellness Approach (the 3 R's: Relapse, rehabilitation and recovery). 1998. Psychiatric Rehabilitation Nurses, Inc. 12204 W. Sunridge Drive. Nine Mile Falls, WA. 99026.
4. Wyandot Mental Health Center. 1223 Meadowlark Lane. Kansas City, Kansas. 66102. 913-287-0007. Contact person: Leslie Young, Director.
5. University of Kansas School of Social Welfare. Twente Hall, Lawrence, Kansas. Consumers As Providers Program. Contact: Diane McDiarmid 785-864-4720.
6. Rapp, C. (1998). The strengths model: Case management with people suffering from severe and persistent mental illness. New York: Oxford University Press.

PART TWO:
PHILOSOPHICAL PERSPECTIVES

Life Experience Is Not a Disease
or Why Medicalizing Madness
Is Counterproductive to Recovery

Juli McGruder, PhD, OTR/L

SUMMARY. The author draws on her personal experience as the family member of an individual with mental illness, on her anthropological research and on that of others to argue that medicalizing madness can be counterproductive to recovery. The medical model is sometimes used in a way that strips away the meaning of the illness experience. Analogies drawn to diseases do not help the understanding of mental illness. Psychiatry is a social practice embedded in a social milieu and that renders it less than objective. It is useful to recognize that the experiences called symptoms have meaning and may have positive and pleasurable aspects. *[Article copies available for a fee from The Haworth Document Delivery Service: 1-800-HAWORTH. E-mail address: <getinfo@*

Juli McGruder is Professor, Occupational Therapy Department, University of Puget Sound, Tacoma, WA.

[Haworth co-indexing entry note]: "Life Experience Is Not a Disease or Why Medicalizing Madness Is Counterproductive to Recovery." McGruder, Juli. Co-published simultaneously in *Occupational Therapy in Mental Health* (The Haworth Press, Inc.) Vol. 17, No. 3/4, 2001, pp. 59-80; and: *Recovery and Wellness: Models of Hope and Empowerment for People with Mental Illness* (ed: Catana Brown) The Haworth Press, Inc., 2001, pp. 59-80. Single or multiple copies of this article are available for a fee from The Haworth Document Delivery Service [1-800-HAWORTH, 9:00 a.m. - 5:00 p.m. (EST). E-mail address: getinfo@haworthpressinc.com].

59

KEYWORDS. Medical model, recovery, madness, positivism, anthropology

I have been asked to write an essay about how the medicalization of madness risks, or may even insure, our turning away from important social phenomena that are an integral part of the labeling or construction of aberrant thought and behavior. Because I believe that everything can be better understood by understanding its history, I elect, first, to tell the reader some of my history both to situate my ideas in the context of a life and to establish my credibility in the readers' eyes. After all, if medical neuroscience holds the key to understanding mental illness, then there is no reason to read my arguments against that view unless my insights are derived from a set of experiences that informs an opinion worth reading.

The social power to define and categorize another person's experience is not a power to be ignored. I hope to convince readers that, in order to support persons who are trying to recover, we must attend to the fullness of their experiences, and not be distracted by their medical diagnoses.

TESTAMENT

I was attracted, as an adolescent, to consider occupational therapy as a career when I saw intriguing paintings at a mental hospital. During that same period I was being taken to counselors and psychologists against my will. My behavior of dating outside my race was seen as pathological by some. I was threatened with incarceration to extract compliance with parental rulings on race relations. It was a long time ago. We have all forgiven each other.

I married outside my race. I became an occupational therapist. I worked for a time in a large state mental hospital. Later I changed practice arenas. Eventually I became an educator and taught mental health courses and neurorehabilitation courses to occupational therapy students. I used a sabbatical from teaching to work in a mental hospital in Africa and do some research comparing ideas on mental illness derived from different OT frames of reference (Evans, 1992a). More interesting than those comparisons was the local view of mental illness as spirit caused (Evans, 1992b). Back in the States, I continued university teaching and began to study socio-cultural anthropology. I have returned many times to the islands of Zanzibar, Tanzania and the mental hospital there. For my doctoral dissertation research in anthropology, I worked with several families that included people diagnosed with schizophrenia. Three families with five people so diagnosed with a collective psychiatric history of 123 years, which I read about in their hospital files, participated in my study. I have been acquainted with one of the families for more than 12 years now. In addition, I did dozens of hours of interview with other persons diagnosed with schizophrenia and with their families. In all I have spent more than two years doing anthropological fieldwork.

Here in the U.S. I have had other formative experiences with psychiatry. As part of my research preparation, I attended a consumer and family education course at a local mental health center. At the same center I attended consumer and family support groups. For 11 years now, I have been the guardian for an elderly woman diagnosed with paranoid schizophrenia. For about two decades I have read, and required my students to read, first person, family and close third person accounts of mental illness. I value these writers' insights.

None of the experiences listed above compares with the education I got last year when a beloved family member went missing for a time, could not sleep, behaved very erratically, laughed, cried and could not explain what was happening to him. I called the local authorities and gave them information that resulted in his involuntary commitment. I knew the law. I knew what the result of my actions would be. That is, I knew I could get him admitted to a psychiatric facility. I wrongly assumed I could also get him out. The day after admission, after some sleep induced by antihistamines but with no other medication, my loved one was calm and coherent. I wanted to take him home from the psychiatric ward and follow up with an outside physician. He was afraid to be there and wanted to come home. We struggled verbally with doctors, lawyers and a judge but lost, despite logical articulate discourse and knowledge of the law. The judge, in particular, seemed only to see a black male criminal in front of him (a hallucination on his part) and assumed the problem to have been street drug induced. (It was not.) "Has there been a toxicology screen?" he insistently and repeatedly asked the treating physician. My relative could not regain his freedom until he agreed to swallow a week's worth of Lithium.

I will draw on all of these learning experiences to argue that people with deviant mental content, disturbing behavior, or unusual beliefs about the nature of reality are not well served by the current positivistic tunnel vision of our biomedical culture that sees all of these problems as biochemical products of an abnormal nervous system. I will argue this based on three interrelated points:

1. The meaning and moral value of behavior can be avoided or stripped away by the processes of biomedical psychiatry that constitute madness as a disease and this is destructive of persons who are trying to recover. Moreover, currently popular disease analogies are inadequate for understanding the experience of mental illness.
2. The "science" of psychiatric diagnosis and treatment is neither objective, nor neutral nor value free. Rather, it is a social process open to bias and influenced by the larger social, political and cultural milieu.
3. Aspects of psychotic experience can be ego-syntonic. The intense and intensely personal experience of psychosis may be pleasurable at times. First person accounts document positive aspects of the experience.

The Meaning and Moral Value of "Symptoms" in the Shared Social World

In *Mirrors of Madness,* Luske documents the struggle between residents in a small community psychiatric facility and the staff who work there over the meaning of the residents' ideas and actions. For example, one resident, Vern, "has insisted all along that his experiences are of a religious nature and in no way indicative of mental illness," despite readily admitting "that psychic pain attends his spiritual quest" (Luske, 1990, p. 97). Other residents speak of what has happened to them in more political terms. Regardless, staff respond by relentlessly labeling residents' experiences as symptoms of a neurobiological disease. They deploy this disease model to insist on compliance with the state requirement that residents in such facilities take medication.

In recent work on questions of human suffering and interpersonal trauma, Kleinman (1999) explored the ways in which human actions transduce meaning and value between social and psychophysiological processes. He argued for the essential inextricability of the moral and the emotional, connected to each other through the body. In other words, the body is a two-way conduit with which human actors both make moral and social sense of bodily processes and physically embody emotions evoked by social experience and ideas about morality. The meaning of acts cannot be derived in isolation from either the social or from the psychophysical. The meaning is created with the act by the actor. The action stands between the world of the body and the social world and makes sense of both.

The acts and ideas that we call symptoms of mental illness are social actions that both create meaning from psychophysiological processes in the body *and* act out social-emotional processes in a bodily way. For example, it is neither a meaningless accident nor a biological imperative that people who experience the high moods of mania often spend money exorbitantly. The consumerist cultural surround and the physiological rush of energy and good feeling come together inside the individual human to make the behavior of buying unneeded expensive things seem entirely apt.

The biological reasoning of today's psychiatry leads us toward a chicken-and-egg kind of questioning about whether the physiology of high mood drives the behavior of spending or the spending elevates mood. These are not useful questions. What is more important is that the spending gives the high mood a social meaning, because consumer goods are given the power of fetish objects in our culture. The social meaning of high-priced objects is tied to highly valued emotions of love of self and signficant others by the thousands of ritualized acts of gift exchange in our culture.

Similarly, it is no accident that when one is filled with an unusual, difficult to interpret feeling of being very different and quite special, one's social surround will interact with that bodily and emotional feeling to shape an interpretation like: "They are watching me and may want to harm me" or "I am a special messenger with an important purpose that will be revealed." When humans voice, or act on, those created meanings, they may be labeled "paranoid" or "grandiose." When one encounters repeated defeats and emotional pain, one may assign the social-emotional meaning to these experiences that the self is not worthy to live or to continue to exist in its present form. Skin cutting, suicide, and catatonia are explained as too much of this or too little of that neurotransmitter, but they are social moral acts. I would hazard a guess that during periods of social history when young women's naked skins were not the cultural fetish objects they are now, young women feeling psychic pain less often expressed it by cutting their skin.

Kleinman's use of "moral" is not a narrow one, nor is it exclusively to do with religious views of right and wrong. Rather, Kleinman noted, social practices are "organized around things that really matter, things that are at stake to participants" (1999, p. 29) and, in that sense, all social activity is concerned with "local moral worlds" (p. 30). While the ideas or actions at stake vary from place to place, the fact that something is at stake is universal. Moreover, knowing what matters also reveals to us what is devalued and what is dangerous to or threatens that which is held to be good and right. Socially organized words, gestures, symbols and actions move meaning and feeling inside each of us and are the stuff of interactions among human actors in the spaces we share with others. The role that biology plays, in this view, is as a malleable under layer that allows rather than constrains the making of meaning and the assignment of moral worth to actions, ideas and emotions.

> Biology is involved, doubtless, but it is made over in the interaction of cultural processes and that is how biology plays its role in human conditions, not as an objectivized essential human nature, but far differently as part of the variety of human conditions. (Kleinman, 1999, p. 29; cf. Kleinman & Becker, 1998)

Clearly the social actors in Luske's ethnography are engaged in a struggle over whether a biological or a social, political or moral frame will be applied to the understanding of individual human experiences. If we apply Kleinman's ideas to current practices in psychoeducation, we can see that discursive practices obscure or deny cultural moral realities. What we say about mental illness reveals what we value and what we fear.

It is quite common in psychoeducation to draw an analogy between serious mental disorders (schizophrenia, bipolar disorders, depression) and conditions which afflict better understood organs and physiological processes (diabetes, hypertension, cardiac conditions) (cf. Moller & Wer, 1993). The thrust of the analogy is, of course, to convince participants that in order to manage their psychiatric disorders they must commit to regular ingestion of medication. It reveals our hope for medical control of differences in mentation. I don't think that the writers and users of such analogies believe them entirely themselves. Still, the persistent use of this kind of analogy foregrounds what is *not* being said. Schizophrenia will never be like diabetes, because the difference in moral value between having a different view of social reality or an unusual set of sensory experiences and having a different level of blood glucose is simply unbreachable. Having palpitations or an arrhythmia does not threaten others in the social surround.

In bringing up threat, I am not here raising the issue of dangerous behavior on the part of some who might be diagnosed with mental illness. Rather, I am speaking here of the existence of a different relationship to the commonly accepted version of reality. The public fears mad persons. I believe that this is not only for their occasional but overrated and over-publicized physical dangerousness–a statistically small threat. Instead, I find that mental illness is feared and has such a stigma because it represents a reversal of what Western humans, in the last few hundred years, have come to value as the essence of human nature. Because our culture so highly values a certain unitariness of consciousness and an illusion of self-control and control of circumstance, we become abject when contemplating mentation that seems more changeable, less restrained and less controllable, more open to outside influence, than we imagine our own to be. Mental illness seems to have less stigma in places, like Zanzibar, where it is widely believed that spirits may take control of human bodies and that all illness, adversity and misfortune are a normal part of human existence programmed by the Almighty. That is, when humans do not assume they have rather complete control of their experiences, they do not so deeply fear those who appear to have lost it.

In psychiatric practice, it is too often the case that once a person's verbal statement of experience or belief can be classified in the nosology of the Diagnostic and Statistical Manual, it is no longer attended to. In the local moral world of psychiatric practice, symptoms have value and utility in their ability to point to a diagnostic label and, thus, to a likely class of medications. In fact, some textbooks teach that delusional material elicited during conversation should be ignored to the extent possible (cf. Kaplan & Sadock, p. 519). I used to teach that principle of "therapeutic interaction" myself. "Don't argue with delusions for they will become more entrenched," I would tell my students, "but don't engage with them at all if you can avoid it. Change the subject. Direct the patient back to the task at hand. State your version of reality and then go on." This advice is *very* different from that given by people who have experienced mental illness themselves. Dr. Frederick Frese (psychologist and person with schizophrenia/mental health consumer) counsels his audience repeatedly that an appropriate response to delusional material would be: "How very interesting. Tell me more" (Frese, 1991). I have changed my advice to students based on this and similar views of therapeutic use of self (cf. Havens & Weiden, 1994).

One standard psychiatry textbook I use has 32 index entries on definitions and nosological utility of different types of delusions and a single one on how one might treat them therapeutically (Kaplan & Sadock, 1998). When attention to the person's subjective experience serves primarily to solve the puzzle of what diagnosis will best fit, more than to achieve an intersubjective understanding of what it is like to live his or her life, the meaning and moral value of that life is demeaned and diminished.

Imagine for a moment that you have felt, for some reason or another, that you have been singled out for some special recognition, or gift, or even threat, and that this experience has dominated your life for some time, motivates much of your behavior, is integral to who you are now. Because of this you get into some trouble. People who say they are there to help you listen once each as you tell your story but then no longer want you to say a word about it or allude to it as the motivator of your actions. Yet to you it is important and explains much of what has happened to you, perhaps including your contact with these ostensible helpers. Recovery from mental illness, sources emphasize, is not synonymous with symptom reduction or eradication (Anthony, 1993). Getting rid of ideas we deem delusional or sensory experience we feel is hallucinatory may not be the help that is needed or desired. Rather, helping consumers recover demands an attention to their stories from their own points of view. In fairness to published psychiatry texts, I must note that they also often advocate, when working with delusions, that therapists voice empathy for the emotional aspect of the consumer's experience. That is, they recommend, for example, saying to the person who feels persecuted: "That must be exhausting." "That must be very frightening." Still, getting that empathic statement right necessitates really listening and being present to hear all about an experience which may shake the roots of one's own local moral world.

I am moved by John Modrow's first person account of mental illness, *How to Become a Schizophrenic,* in which he wrote:

> I cannot think of anything more destructive of one's sense of worth as a human being than to believe that the inner core of one's being is sick–that one's thoughts, values, feelings, and beliefs are merely the meaningless symptoms of a sick mind. Undoubtedly the single most important causal factor behind my mental breakdown was a sense of worth so badly shaken that not even the most florid delusions of grandeur could save it. What the concept of "mental illness" offered me was "scientific proof" that I was utterly worth-

less, and would always be worthless. It was just the nature of my genes, chemistry and brain processes–something I could do nothing about. (1992, p. 147)

Similarly, Sally Clay, in addressing the First National Forum on Recovery from Mental Illness, said:

Those of us who have had the experience called "mental illness" know in our hearts that something profound is missing in these diagnoses. They do not take into account what we have actually endured. Even if the "bad" chemical or the "defective" gene is someday found, madness has its own reality that demands attention. (1994)

Jay Neugeboren wrote about the experiences of his brother, Robert, who is diagnosed with chronic schizophrenia, and suggested that the notion of "no-fault brain diseases" is absurd. Neugeboren argued against the "dead-end scientific materialism that would reduce Robert to a flawed heretical biological inheritance that somehow determines his behavior and his fate" (1997, p. 302), and asked the following rhetorical questions about what would become of Robert if medication eradicated his symptoms at this point:

What does he do with his history? What does he do with his memories, doubts, habits, and fears? The sad truth is that who he is–his identity as Robert Neugeboren and nobody else, a human being forever in process, forever growing, changing and evolving–is made up, to this point in time, largely of what most of us have come to call his illness. And if he gives that up, as it were–if he denies that this so-called illness is central to his life and being (and if he merely *fixes* his symptoms instead of understanding their causes), and does not hold on to his illness and its history as a legitimate, real and unique part of his ongoing self–what of him, at fifty two years old, will be left? (1997, p. 303, emphasis in the original)

Increasingly, mental health professionals have embraced a neurobiological view of schizophrenia and some of us have done so because it seemed this view would eventually destigmatize the disorder; would someday make it just like diabetes and hypertension. Here, Modrow, Clay and Neugeboren tell us that it is simply not so. Moreover, seeing oneself as having a "brain disease" may not facilitate recovery at all, as it did not for Modrow. Instead, resisting this view energized his recovery. Deegan also emphasizes that "accepting that one has an illness is not a necessary part of the recovery process" (1998, p. 2).

Of all the precepts of the recovery movement, the disjuncture between the disease model with symptom eradication via psychotropic drugs and recovery as a social and psychological journey may be the most important and yet, perhaps, the most difficult for health professionals to accept. It is not *necessary* to the practice of psychiatry to ignore the meaning and moral value of symptoms in the shared social world. Yet, it appears quite possible to practice psychiatry and psychiatric occupational therapy in just that way. I think that too often we practice as if blinkered by the exigencies of the medical model, and that practicing in this way endangers consumers' recovery processes. I urge us to pay attention to the meanings of symptoms from the client's perspective, not in some Freudian sense of assigning meaning based on unconscious symbolization, but to the moral meaning that recovering individuals invest them with, in the contexts of their life experiences. While systems of symbolization like Freud's or Jung's that posit some universalistic meaning based on a unified culture may hold useful clues, more contemporary ideas about cultural variation demand recognition that symbols may be quite personal and idiosyncratic or may be shared by a subcultural group this is embedded in and actively resists the dominant culture.

Social, Political and Cultural Influence on Psychiatric Practice

Since we heard for years about the political uses of psychiatry in the Soviet Union, it should not be hard for us to believe that politics influences the practice of psychiatry. Some, however, will be loathe to accept such influences as operational in our own society. Yet biomedical psychiatry, for all of its scientific trappings, is practiced by fallible humans who live in a cultural surround in which politics, economics and history are forces that affect our judgment and color the way we see other humans. Psychiatric health professionals are as prone to bias and stereotypical thinking as other citizens.

Perhaps the clearest way to prove that social biases affect psychiatric processes is to point to the body of literature on misdiagnosis of African Americans. Studies from the 1970s to the 1990s reveal a tendency toward overdiagnosis of schizophrenia and underdiagnosis of mood disorders in African Americans. Epidemiological studies (Adebimpe,1981a, 1981b; Bell & Metha; 1980, 1981; Coleman & Baker, 1994; Jones &

Gray, 1986) and experimental attributions research (Loring & Powell, 1988) show that–symptom profiles being equal–people of color are more likely to get more severe, less hopeful diagnostic labels (e.g., schizophrenia over bipolar disorder). Images of Africans as savage, out of control and mentally deficient have a long history in our popular culture and mass media (Riggs, 1986). These images are so engrained in our culture that many people are not cognizant that their negative effects persist. In comparison with European Americans, African Americans were more likely to be involuntarily committed (Lindsey & Paul, 1989), to receive drugs more frequently and receive larger doses of stronger drugs, to experience more use of restraints and seclusion and to be referred less frequently for occupational and recreational therapy (Bond, DiCandia & McKinnon, 1988; Flaherty & Meager, 1980; Psychiatric News, 1984).

The act of declaring another human being to be dangerous to himself or others and to have a mental disorder is a political act. It is a legal act that allows for the use of force to extract compliance with treatment that years from now may seem just as evil and absurd as rotating chairs, lobotomy and wet packs do to most of us now. The speech act of diagnosis is also a medical act, but it is not in the same realm as the diagnosing of other medical disorders. It is certainly not neutral or value free. As Rhodes has observed:

> Medicine, because of its bias toward the uncovering of natural facts, represents the body in ways that are powerfully suggestive of a natural reality separate from the social . . . The effect, if not the intention, is to make the social invisible, and to place the sickness, as a natural process or entity, inside the individual . . . By placing the body and bodily experience in the realm of nature, biomedicine conceals both the social causes of sickness and the social embeddedness of the experience of sickness. (1990, pp. 167-168)

> Biomedical theory and practice is problematic and not simply when it fails to address cultural and social issues involved in individual patient care but because of its embeddedness and (often) sustaining role in dominant political and economic systems. (1990, p. 172)

Even if we firmly believe that DSM diagnoses and psychotropic drugs are an important part of treatment, we might temper our enthusiasm for them by admitting that they are not produced in a vacuum.

Rather they are developed and produced in a social milieu that is (1) given to imbuing reductionistic explanations of human behavior with more power than more macro level social explanations have (Gelman, 1999) and (2) built on a capitalistic economic base (Luske, 1990). We might begin by acknowledging that much research on mental illness is conducted by large pharmaceutical corporations with a vested interest in selling drugs as adequate treatment. We might admit that psychopharmaceutical treatments for "brain diseases" are pre-eminent not because they are the exclusive remedies for biological problems we clearly understand, but because more money is spent establishing them than investigating or establishing any other sort of treatment. Sales of psychotropic drugs turn huge profits. We might note that advertisement of mass-produced drugs, of both the therapeutic and recreational varieties, is clearly a gendered practice in our culture in its reproduction of stereotypical sex roles. For example, one will see two or three commercials for anti-depressants and anti-anxiety medications during Oprah or a Lifetime channel movie, but none during an NFL or NBA game, during which beer is advertised instead. Some people in our society are simply more frequently seen as ill or defective, by virtue of their race or gender, and, as we shall see below, some are more likely to accept an illness label for themselves. Others are forced or inveigled or relentlessly pressed to do so. Finally, we might admit that almost since their inception the efficacy and necessity of the medications now called by the misnomer "anti-psychotics" has been overstated and oversold. (For a convincing and very detailed argument on this last point, see *Medicating Schizophrenia: A History* by Sheldon Gelman, 1999.)

When Rhodes (1984) examined the talk of psychiatric staff and patients about medication issues, she found their discourse marked by metaphor that could persuade, and could communicate experience or expectation, but that, just as often, confused each other and entangled issues. Rhodes found that communication about medication was most successfully managed by those who were willing to adopt the point of view and idioms of the person with whom they were conversing. Thus, patients got clinicians to listen by speaking in medical metaphors that were distant from their actual bodily experiences of the drugs. Staff elicited better cooperation from patients by speaking about medication effects in ways that were closer to the patients' experience of it. Metaphor was deployed–successfully by some, unsuccessfully by others–to bridge the crucial gap between the experiences of taking medication and of giving medication, and participants' senses of identity around those experiences. This discrepant experience and the inadequacies of language for communicating about it cannot be ignored when we try to assist individuals toward recovery.

If we cannot acknowledge that the consumer is often recovering not only from the effects of mental illness but also from the effects of its diagnosis and treatment, then we will have difficulty forging alliances with recovering individuals. I urge us to be critical observers of the systems of care in which we are complicit, as workers or simply as citizens. Crepeau (2000) and Luske (1990) showed how patients who don't comply with role expectations of health care workers challenge their belief systems and provoke discomfort and frustration. Such emotional reactions, while expectable, may motivate a countertherapeutic retaliation against the patient. Crepeau pointed out, however, that frustration need not be handled this way but could be used to fuel renewed efforts at understanding the patient. Like Kleinman, Crepeau saw moral qualities inherent in staff-patient and staff-staff interactions. She clearly described the struggle for moral authority embedded in narrative construction of what was going on in patients' lives. I agree with Crepeau that in order to promote humanistic psychiatric practice we could challenge and question the moral dimensions of our re-constructions of patients' experiences.

Estroff et al. (1991) examined 169 informants' own constructions of identity and ideas about illness in the face of diagnosis with a major psychiatric disorder, following each for a two year period. I will summarize her findings in some detail. Estroff's unique study provides good food for thought about how the social milieu affects the process by which someone newly diagnosed with a mental disorder might incorporate that information into statements about his or her identity. Estroff found that her participants' illness accounts and self-labels were mutable and situational. Social processes, such as hospitalization and inclusion or exclusion from the family home, had a great deal to do with self-generated illness accounts and identity labels. Nowhere was the impact of social processes more observable than in Estroff's material on race and gender.

Race and gender factors interacted with the social processes of institutionalization and could facilitate acceptance of a disease label or energize reaction against it. Noting a proportion of African American men in her sample greater than their proportion in the general population, Estroff commented on the tendency to overdiagnose schizophrenia in African Americans. During the initial interviews African American men were the least likely of all groups to accept an illness label, while European American men in Estroff's sample tended to identify with authority figures and accept psychiatric labels more readily. African American women and European American women were more similar to one another in their proportions of accepting or resisting disease labels, and in accounts of the causes of illness. Their odds of accepting a diagnostic label were intermediate between those of European and African American men. Overall, however, European Americans of both genders made more statements that reflected belief in medical or clinical causes for their problems while African Americans used a broader range of kinds of ideas to account for their difficulties, including more social and more spiritual explanations.

Over the illness course studied, African American men typically continued to resist diagnostic labels and European American men gradually distanced themselves from such labels. Over time, more European American women in the study labeled themselves as mentally ill while the proportion of African American women who would accept such a label for themselves remained consistent at about 37%. Resistance to authority may have been part of a habitual self-preserving strategy in a hostile environment for African Americans. Estroff (1991) also remarked that several of the African American male participants appeared to have been misdiagnosed. If so, this resistance strategy was certainly adaptive. (See Whaley, 1998, for insights on the adaptive utility of some behaviors labeled as symptoms.)

Estroff noted that interviews with participants of both genders and races elicited a great deal of talk about the ways in which the participants were just like other people. Their difficulties and reactions were perceived by themselves as essentially "normal" or on a continuum with other kinds of problems experienced by other people. Estroff and colleagues drew this important lesson:

> The enormous amount of normalizing talk we elicited was at times defiant, urgent, plaintive, and even whimsical. Regardless of tone, this kind of discourse was always meant to persuade us, and no doubt our informants themselves, that whether mentally ill or not, the individual was worthwhile, one of us–normal. Perhaps chronicity and disability begin when normalizing talk ends, or when the individual thinks no one is listening. One compelling challenge for anthropologists and clinicians alike is to keep the conversation going. (1991, p. 363)

I think we can best help with the recovery process by listening and resisting any need we may feel to enforce acceptance of clinical medical etiologies as this may have the effect of turning off the conversation or truncating the exploratory journey in identity reconstruction that, perforce, follows psychiatric hospitalization. Respectful listening without labeling, admitting that psychiatry is a social practice open to bias and tempering our enthusiasm for drugs as part of treatment can go a long way toward establishing ourselves as allies in recovery.

The Positive Aspects of Psychotic Experience

As health professionals we tend to think of mental illnesses as afflictions that overwhelm the normal aspects of consumers' lives and cause them to suffer. There is, of course, some truth to that view. We tend to ignore or de-emphasize the enjoyment people may feel in the heightened states of energy or awareness that precede or accompany a psychotic break with ordinary reality. For the most part we lack, in the industrialized West, a cultural way to valorize or honor such experience. Although there are some religious enclaves in America that value ecstatic experience, when their meager power comes up against that of psychiatry, medical power wins. This was certainly the case for an African American friend of mine whose prayer group came to the ward to pray with her during a psychiatric confinement. When several group members including "the patient" were moved by the spirit to speak in tongues, and act upon ecstatic feelings in other ways, the medical director banned subsequent prayer circles.

Many first person accounts, some recent and some older, attest to the fact that the experience of psychosis may be ego-syntonic and the person involved in it may undertake certain actions to enhance or amplify it. (This seems especially true in the early stages but is not limited to that time.) The thesis of Podvoll's book *The Seduction of Madness* is exactly this: that there is agency involved in pursuit of hallucinatory experience. Based on clinical experience and on the journals of people undergoing psychotic experience, Podvoll described the kinds of actions people may take: doing without sleep, entertaining repetitive problems or thought courses, experiments with movement. He also described the qualities of such experiences that slip out of control of the active seeker.

Frese (1992) spoke about pleasures of his mystical experience "cruising the cosmos," but also noted that the process is quite hard to control and can become frightening. He argued that productive creativity can spring from "poetic logic." Modrow wrote about things he did to heighten the unusual feeling state that bloomed into psychosis; things like walking late at night along lonely roads and staring into the lights of oncoming cars. He recounted the magnificence of the feeling he had for the time that he perceived himself as John the Baptist reincarnate.

Mark Vonnegut in *The Eden Express* wrote of experiencing small co-incidences (e.g., pulling the right change from his pocket without try-ing) as signs of living in a state of grace and actively seeking to remain open to these small gifts from God (p. 28, 29 and passim). States of grace were usually accompanied by "a sensual rush of warmth and well-being" (p. 29). Vonnegut also described holding still and straining to hear the voices, some hostile, but many pleasant, warm and loving, bringing answers to puzzling questions (p. 106). About his first visual hallucination he wrote:

> When I first saw the face coming toward me I had thought, "Oh goody." What I had in mind was a nice reasonable conversation. I had lots of things I wanted to talk about, lots of questions it must have answers to. God, Jesus, the Bible, the Ching, mescaline, art, music, history, evolution, physics, mathematics. How they all fit together. Just a nice bull session, but a bull session with a differ-ence. A bull session with someone who *knew*. (pp. 74-75, empha-sis in the original)

Ecstatic sexual feelings in the absence of physical sexual activity were another positive side of Vonnegut's early schizophrenic experi-ence.

> I was electric with sexuality. Breathing gave me orgasm upon or-gasm. I can't begin to describe what dancing with angels was like. Occasionally the puritan in me would try to worry about having to pay for this someday, but the pleasure was so all-engulfing there was very little room for second thoughts. (p. 109)

In *An Unquiet Mind,* Jamison related the wistful sadness she still feels upon seeing any representation of the planet Saturn, now that her moods are regulated with medication. During periods of manic mood she had felt herself

> . . . gliding, flying, now and again lurching through cloud banks and ethers, past stars and across fields of ice crystals. Even now I can see in my mind's rather peculiar eye an extraordinary shatter-ing and shifting of light; inconsistent but ravishing colors laid out

across miles of circling rings; and the almost imperceptible, some-what surprisingly pallid moons of this Catherine wheel of a planet. I remember singing "Fly Me to the Moons," as I swept past those of Saturn and thinking myself terribly funny. (1995, p. 90)

A celebrated American poet, H. D. (aka Hilda Doolittle, 1886-1961), companion of Ezra Pound, D. H. Lawrence, T. S. Elliot, William Carlos Williams, an adventurous woman who suffered several "breakdowns," is another fascinating source of insight into hallucinatory experience. She engaged with Freud as his partner in her own analysis; he consid-ered her a friend. Books she wrote during her analysis celebrate her childhood ability to do what we might clinically label dissolving or sus-pending her ego boundaries (*The Gift, HERmione*). Her gift–a feeling of merging with nature, trees, landscapes, and other people–powered her early "imagist" poetry. In her analysis with Freud, documented in her book *Tribute to Freud* (1956), she shared visions that she experienced during her travels: picture writing on the wall in her room in Greece, an apparition of a man she saw on board ship. In the following passage it is easy to see how, like Vonnegut, she expected important insights and so-lutions to artistic problems from these visions and yet how she was con-strained in her pursuit of them by fear that they were "symptoms." The visions themselves, the process of describing the visions in writing and her writing to describe herself relating the visions to Freud, are all en-twined in her account. This passage follows her description of three fig-ures she saw form on the wall, and her description of them to Freud:

So far, so good–or so far so dangerous, so abnormal a "symptom." At least the writing is consistent . . . But here I pause or the hand pauses–it is as if there were a slight question as to the conclusion or the direction of the symbols. I mean, it was as if a painter had stepped back from a canvas the better to regard the composition of the picture, or a musician had paused at the music stand for a mo-ment . . . That is in myself too, a wonder at the seemliness, or safety even, of continuing this experience or this experiment. (1956, pp. 46-47)

She sought reassurance while watching the visions from her close fe-male friend and companion, Bryher:

I can turn now to her, though I do not budge an inch or break the sustained crystal gazing stare at the wall before me. I say to

Bryher, "There have been pictures here–I thought they were shadows at first, but they are light, not shadow. They are quite simple objects–but of course it's very strange. I can break away from them now if I want–it's just a matter of concentrating–what do you think? Shall I stop? Shall I go on?" (1956, p. 47)

Her friend advised her to go on. She did:

Yet although now assured of her support, my own head is splitting with the ache of concentration. I know that if I let go, lessen the intensity of my stare and shut my eyes or even blink my eyes, to rest them, the pictures will fade out. My curiosity is insatiable. This has never happened to me before, it may never happen again. (1956, p. 49)

What is most apparent in H. D.'s account, and in the other first person accounts, is the intentionality, the active agency of the seer of visions or hearer of voices. Moreover, the sensory experiences are rich with meaning and import for the agent who pursues them. Here we have come full circle in my argument and can see how the third point relates back to the first. Things that we might call "symptoms" are not only ego-syntonic at times, but meaningful and important to those who experience them. If our treatment is to be helpful to recovery, we must recognize that.

I was delighted to learn in the process of doing some research for this essay that hearers of voices have organized in Europe, as the Hearing Voices Network (cf. Thomas, 1997; Romme & Escher, 1993) A Dutch psychiatrist and consumer were originators of this new and "emancipatory" approach to unusual perceptual experience. After an appearance on a TV talk show that netted them 450 interested callers who heard voices, they undertook a survey of ways that people coped with or managed the experience (Romme & Escher, 1993). Results of the survey indicate that the single most important contributor to success in employing coping strategies was a supportive social environment. This is most significant in that the coping strategies reported often involved actively engaging in selectively listening and responding to the voices, during periods of time set aside for that purpose. These active engagement strategies were reported as much more successful than strategies of ignoring or distracting. Some reported trying out the interpretation of the auditory experience by asking themselves questions like: "If this voice comes from some aspect of myself, what is it that I should be taking from it? What is it trying to tell me? What lesson is there to be learned?

What might this say about how I am feeling?" In my own conversations with two women–one here in the States, one in Zanzibar–I have heard about the utility of the strategy of arguing with and talking back to critical voices, asserting another perspective. Both women told me that they tried to counter criticisms silently, but were often only able to silence the heard voices by raising their own.

A conference followed Romme and Escher's survey and the organization of groups followed that (Thomas, 1997). Hearing Voices Network provides a model of a successful, consumer-driven recovery movement that explicitly removes something considered a nearly pathognomonic symptom of schizophrenia from its biomedical psychiatric context and instead normalizes it.

CONCLUSION

Thinking about the Hearing Voices Network helps me tie together the three points I've raised against our entrapment in a medical epistemology for viewing madness. As Romme and Escher concluded: "We may therefore view the hearing of voices not solely as a discrete individual psychological experience but as an interactional phenomenon reflecting the nature of the individual's relationship to his or her own environment" (1993, p. 16). That is, to revisit my first point, things that are called symptoms have meaning and value in the shared social world and if we want to help people recover we should honor and not ignore that. Using biomedicine as the frame of reference for viewing such problems easily lends itself to ignoring the meaningfulness, import and moral value of individual experience. We might employ biomedicine as a partial frame, useful at times, but incomplete and inadequate for much of what we want to accomplish. I am certain from my work in Zanzibar that it is not necessary for families or others in the consumers' social-emotional surround to accept the language of disordered brain, chemical imbalances and defective genes in order to give love and support in ways that help. In fact, some of my observations from Zanzibar lead me to believe that socializing families into the biomedical frame for viewing their loved ones may do more harm than good (McGruder, 1998).

That we ought to adopt a critical stance toward the social processes that comprise psychiatric diagnosis and treatment was my second point. We can be willing to interrogate psychiatric practices that reflect social ills–like racism, sexism, and class bias–that exist in the society at large.

This too requires a willingness to let go of the positivism of psychiatric medicine, however hopeful or promising we may have found it. If we deny the social and political aspects of what happens to "consumers" forced to accept treatment against their wills, or even cajoled into accepting medication that makes them feel miserable, we do a certain violence–or at minimum give disrespect–to their experiences. (The very irony of the now popular term "consumer" of mental health services cannot go unremarked, when so many have literally no choice of health care provider or facility–let alone whether to be treated or not–and hence no real consumer power.) Like Estroff, we can support the identity reconstruction that people undertake after psychosis by listening to whatever explanations are meaningful and make moral sense in their worlds.

In so doing–my last point–we can begin to see that the things we think of as "symptoms" are not all bad and may give a life journey meaning. There are sufficient hints in first person accounts to suggest that one of the negative aspects of hallucinatory experience is the anxiety caused by the negative social labeling of this state as mad and bad. For some the experience itself is not frightening. The fear and anxiety come in knowing how this experience will be evaluated by others who have not had it. Seeing that "symptoms" may be pleasurable and meaningful and need not be relentlessly eradicated in order to control a "disease" lays the foundation for an approach to consumers that is more conducive to empathic partnering for recovery.

REFERENCES

Adebimpe, V.R. (1981a). Overview: White norms and psychiatric diagnosis of black patients. *American Journal of Psychiatry, 138,* 279-285.

Adebimpe, V.R. (1981b). Hallucinations and delusions in black psychiatric patients. *Journal of the National Medical Association, 73,* 517-520.

Anthony, W.A. (1993). Recovery from mental illness: The guiding vision of the mental health service system in the 1990s. *Psychosocial Rehabilitation Journal, 16,* 11-23.

Bell, C.C. & Metha, H. (1980). The misdiagnosis of black patients with manic depressive illness. *Journal of the National Medical Association, 72,* 141-145.

Bell, C.C. & Metha, H. (1981). The misdiagnosis of black patients with manic depressive illness: Second in a series. *Journal of the National Medical Association, 73,* 101-107.

Bond, C.F., DiCandia C.G., & MacKinnon, J.R. (1988). Responses to violence in a psychiatric setting: The role of the patient's race. *Personality and Social Psychology Bulletin, 14,* 448-458.

Clay, S. (1994) The Wounded Prophet. Paper presented at the First National Forum on Recovery from Mental Illness, National Institute of Mental Health and Ohio Department of Mental Health. April 1994. Unpublished manuscript.

Coleman, D. & Baker, F.M. (1994). Misdiagnosis of schizophrenia among black veterans. *Journal of Nervous and Mental Diseases, 182*, 527-528.

Crepeau, E.B. (2000). Reconstructing Gloria: A narrative analysis of team meetings. *Qualitative Health Research, 10*, 766-787.

Deegan, P.E. (1998) Some principles and themes of the recovery process. Handout from the National Empowerment Center, Inc. Lawrence MA. http://www.power2u.org

Estroff, S.E. with Lachicotte, W.S., Illingworth L.C., & Johnston, A. (1991). Everybody's got a little mental illness: Accounts of illness and self among people with severe, persistent, mental illness. *Medical Anthropology Quarterly, 5*, 331-369.

Evans, J. (1992a). A cross cultural test of the validity of occupational therapy assessments for patients with schizophrenia. *American Journal of Occupational Therapy, 48*, 685-695.

Evans, J. (1992b). Schizophrenia: Living with madness here and in Zanzibar. *Occupational Therapy in Health Care, 8*, 53-71.

Frese, F.J. (1991). Schizophrenia: Surviving in the world of normals. [videotape]. Beachwood, Ohio: Wellness Productions, Inc.

Frese, F.J. (1992). Keynote address and handout, "Twelve aspects of coping skills for seriously mentally ill persons" from the American Occupational Therapy Association, annual conference, Houston.

Gelman, S. (1999). *Medicating Schizophrenia: A history*. New Brunswick, New Jersey: Rutgers University Press.

Havens, L. & Weiden, P. (1994). Psychotherapeutic management techniques in the treatment of outpatients with schizophrenia. *Hospital and Community Psychiatry, 45*, 549-555.

H.D. (Doolittle, Hilda) (1982) *The Gift*. New York: New Directions.

H.D. (Doolittle, Hilda) (1974; original,1956) *Tribute to Freud*. New York: New Directions.

H.D. (Doolittle, Hilda) (1981) *HERmione*. New York: New Directions.

Jamison, K.R. (1996). *An Unquiet Mind*. New York: Random House.

Jones, B.E. & Gray, B.A. (1986). Problems in diagnosing schizophrenia and affective disorders among blacks. *Hospital and Community Psychiatry, 37*, 61-65.

Kaplan, H.I. & Sadock, B. J. (1998). *Kaplan and Sadock's Synopsis of Psychiatry: Behavioral sciences, clinical psychiatry*. (8th ed.). Baltimore: Williams & Wilkins.

Kleinman, A. (1999). From One Human Nature to Many Human Conditions: An anthropological enquiry into suffering as moral experience in a disordering age. *Suomen Antropologi/Journal of the Finnish Anthropological Society, 24*, 23-36.

Kleinman, A. & Becker, A.E. (1998). Sociosomatics–The contribution of anthropology to psychosomatic medicine. *Psychosomatic Medicine, 60*, 389-393.

Lindsey, K.P. & Paul, G.L. (1989). Involuntary commitments to public mental institutions: issues involving the overrepesentation of blacks and assessment of relevant functions. *Psychological Bulletin, 106*, 171-183.

Loring, M. & Powell, B. (1988) Gender, race and DSM II: A study of objectivity of psychiatric diagnostic behavior. *Journal of Health and Social Behavior, 29*, 1-22.

Luske, B. (1990). *Mirrors of Madness: Patrolling the Psychic Border.* New York: Aldine De Gruyter.

McGruder, J. (1999). Madness in Zanzibar: "Schizophrenia" in three families in the "developing" world. Unpublished doctoral dissertation, University of Washington, Department of Anthropology.

Modrow, J. (1992). *How to Become a Schizophrenic: The Case Against Biological Psychiatry.* Everett, Washington: Apollyon Press.

Moller, M. D., & Wer, J. E. (1993). *How to enter the world of psychosis: A family educational perspective.* Nine Mile Falls, Washington: The Center for Patient and Family Mental Health Education.

Neugeboren, J. (1997). *Imagining Robert: My brother, madness and survival.* New York: Henry Holt.

Podvoll, E. (1990). *The seduction of madness.* New York: Harper Collins.

Psychiatric News (no by line) (1984). Blacks more likely to get long acting drugs. *Psychiatric News,* June 15, 1984. pp. 18-19.

Rhodes, L. A. (1984). "This will clear your mind": The use of metaphor for medication in psychiatric settings. *Culture, Medicine and Psychiatry, 8,* 49-70.

Rhodes, L. A. (1990). Studying biomedicine as a cultural system. In Johnson & Sargent (Eds.), *Medical Anthropology* (pp. 160-173). New York: Praeger.

Riggs, M. (1986) "Ethnic Notions." [videorecording] San Francisco: California Newsreels.

Romme, M.A.J. & Escher, A.D. (1993) The new approach: A Dutch experiment. In M.A.J. and A.D. Escher (Eds.). *Accepting Voices.* London: MIND.

Thomas, P. (1997) *The Dialectics of Schizophrenia.* New York: Free Association Books.

Vonnegut, M. (1975) *The Eden Express.* New York: Praeger.

Whaley, A. L. (1998). Cross-Cultural Perspective on Paranoia: A focus on the Black American experience. *Psychiatric Quarterly, 69*(4), 325-343.

Teaching Approaches
and Occupational Therapy Psychoeducation

René Padilla, MS, OTR/L

SUMMARY. Patient education has become an important feature of any treatment program. Psychoeducational procedures dominate the treatment used by occupational therapy practitioners in psychiatric rehabilitation. Occupational therapy literature frequently describes the content of psychoeducational programs but rarely examines the teaching approach therapists use in them. It is necessary, therefore, to begin carefully questioning how we are approaching psychoeducation and justifying it as a method compatible with our basic philosophical principles and our growing understanding of occupation. Three approaches to teaching are examined and contrasted with occupational therapy values: the executive approach, the therapist approach, and the liberationist approach. Each of these approaches points to dramatically different outcomes of the therapeutic process. Ultimately, they bring into question the way in which we build a relationship with our clients. The liberationist approach is proposed as the best guide of how and why to use psychoeducation in the quest for providing authentic occupational therapy. *[Article copies available for a fee from The Haworth Document Delivery Service: 1-800-HAWORTH. E-mail address: <getinfo@ haworthpressinc.com> Website: <http://www.HaworthPress.com> © 2001 by The Haworth Press, Inc. All rights reserved.]*

René Padilla is Chair, Department of Occupational Therapy, School of Pharmacy and Allied Health Professions, Creighton University, 2500 California Plaza, Omaha, NE 68178 (E-mail: Rpadilla@creighton.edu).

[Haworth co-indexing entry note]: "Teaching Approaches and Occupational Therapy Psychoeducation." Padilla, René. Co-published simultaneously in *Occupational Therapy in Mental Health* (The Haworth Press, Inc.) Vol. 17, No. 3/4, 2001, pp. 81-95; and: *Recovery and Wellness: Models of Hope and Empowerment for People with Mental Illness* (ed: Catana Brown) The Haworth Press, Inc., 2001, pp. 81-95. Single or multiple copies of this article are available for a fee from The Haworth Document Delivery Service [1-800-HAWORTH, 9:00 a.m. - 5:00 p.m. (EST). E-mail address: getinfo@haworthpressinc.com].

KEYWORDS. Education, executive approach, therapist approach, liberationist approach

INTRODUCTION

Patient education has become an important feature of any treatment program. In the last two decades the mental health literature has increasingly used the term "psychoeducation" in reference to techniques found useful in the treatment and rehabilitation of patients with severe and persistent mental illness and their families (Spencer et al., 1988; McFarlane, Lukens, & Link, 1995; Pollio, North & Douglas, 1998; Lubin, Loris, Burt & Johnson, 1998). One of the earliest definitions of the term stated that psychoeducation is "the use of educational techniques, methods, and approaches to aid in the recovery from the disabling effects of mental illness or as an adjunct to the treatment of the mentally ill, usually within the framework of another ongoing treatment approach or as part of a research program" (Barter, 1984, p. 23). This definition was further refined by Goldman (1988) who stated that psychoeducation is "education or training of a person with a psychiatric disorder in subject areas that serve the goals of treatment and rehabilitation, for example, enhancing the person's acceptance of his illness, promoting active cooperation with treatment and rehabilitation, and strengthening the coping skills that compensate for deficiencies caused by the disorder" (p. 667).

A basic assumption of psychoeducation is that information can enhance understanding of the illness, needed treatment resources, and supportive services available (Greenberg et al., 1988). Outcomes reported often include increase in daily living skills and adaptive capacities and the creation of more productive alliances between patients, families, and mental health professionals, making treatment more efficient and cost-effective (Dixon, Adams & Lucksted, 2000). Although the specific elements and construction of the various programs vary, all programs have a common characteristic in that they are professionally created and led, often by a multidisciplinary team (Solomon, 1996; Pollio, North & Foster, 1998; Dixon, 1999). These teams frequently include an occupational therapy practitioner (Dixon, 1999).

Psychoeducational procedures dominate the treatment used by occupational therapists in psychiatric rehabilitation (Hayes & Halford, 1993). Emphasis in occupational therapy intervention in mental health is often placed on life skills training through behavioral approaches

(Fine, 1980; Barris, 1985; Bartlow & Hartwig, 1989; Klasson, 1989). Occupational therapy literature frequently describes the content of psychoeducational programs but rarely examines the teaching approach therapists use in them. Presumably, the behavioral emphasis on life skills training is viewed as consistent with basic occupational therapy philosophy, and therefore the teaching methods used are not carefully scrutinized. However, several studies have recently brought into question the generalizability to community life of skills learned in occupational therapy treatment (Wallace et al., 1992; Hayes & Halford, 1993). Of even more concern is the possibility that occupational therapy treatment has no greater relative effectiveness than training provided in psychoeducation by paraprofessionals (Liberman et al., 1998). It is necessary, therefore, to begin carefully questioning how we are approaching psychoeducation and justifying it as a method compatible with our basic philosophical principles and our growin understanding of occupation.

BASIC PRINCIPLE:
THE OCCUPATIONAL NATURE
OF THE HUMAN BEING

In order to evaluate the compatibility of various teaching approaches with occupational therapy, it is necessary to first briefly review some foundational philosophical beliefs of the profession. This review is not intended to be exhaustive, but to highlight general principles that should be present in any and all services we provide in order for them to be recognized as unique to occupational therapy.

A fundamental belief of occupational therapy is that "Man is an active being whose development is influenced by the use of purposeful activity" (American Occupational Therapy Association [AOTA], 1995-a, p. 10). Central to this concept is the human capacity for intrinsic motivation, self initiation and choice (Dickerson, 1996). Yerxa (1967) emphasized that occupational therapy recognizes this notion by supporting the patient's choice of activity, stating that "it is impossible to force any human being to initiate without his choosing to do so; choice is one of the keys to our unique therapeutic process. It is also a necessity if we are to achieve the ultimate goal of occupational therapy, that is, the ability of the person to function in his environment with self-actualization. For no matter how well-conceived the therapeutic program, the resulting achievement of the client's function depends both upon his capacities and his choice to use them" (1967, p. 23). According to Yerxa (1967), the therapeutic process is one in which clients are able to gradually "experience their possibilities" and become increasingly informed about reality in order to make choices for which they can anticipate the results. In this process, clients are able to self-actualize.

From its inception, occupational therapy chose occupation as its unique method to help clients function with self-actualization (AOTA, 1995-b). The term "occupation" has been the subject of debate throughout the history of the profession because of the complexity it represents. Derived from the Latin root "occupaio," meaning "to seize or take possession," occupation conveys action and anticipation (Englehardt, 1977) and the taking of control over one's life (Reilly, 1966). For some, the term refers to the active participation in self-maintenance, work, leisure and play (AOTA, 1993). For others, occupation is synonymous with "purposeful activity" (Henderson et al., 1991). Occupations are also considered to be "the ordinary and familiar things that people do every day" (AOTA, 1995-b, p. 1015). Occupation has been described as the behavior which results from the volitional and adaptive interaction of the human being with the environment (Kielhofner, 1995), and as "a complex dynamic involving individuals and their purposive behavior within environmental contexts that have meaning and which change over time" (Nelson, 1996, p. 775). Occupation has also been explained as self-initiated, goal directed and socially sanctioned daily pursuits which are often personally satisfying and which shape, in part, one's perception of quality of life (Yerxa et al., 1990). Finally, occupation has been recognized as a principal way through which human beings learn to live in community and contribute meaningfully to society (Grady, 1995).

Although a singular definition is elusive, we can summarize here by saying that the term occupation represents the adaptive process through which human beings take charge of their own lives and actively realize their own particular meaning both as individuals and as contributors to their communities. Ultimately, any occupational therapy intervention should contribute to this end (Yerxa, 1966). This, then, is the philosophical filter through which we must examine all therapeutic approaches used in treatment, including educational ones.

APPROACHES TO TEACHING AND OCCUPATIONAL THERAPY PHILOSOPHY

As with occupation, "teaching" is also a multidimensional concept that defies definition. Although there are numerous schools of thought, each with its own set of philosophical values and educational techniques, they can be classified into three very basic and broad approaches to teaching, including the "executive," the "therapist," and the "liberationist" approaches (Fenstermacher & Soltis, 1998). Each of these approaches must be examined in light of psychoeducation and of occupation, the treatment of choice in occupational therapy.

At first glance, each of the teaching approaches is representative of a conception of education that seems compatible with occupational therapy philosophy. Translating them to our work with clients, we might say that the executive conception is that we must shape clients to the current norms and conventions of society. The therapist conception is that we must encourage the development of each client's individual potential. Finally, the liberationist conception is that we must teach clients the knowledge that will focus their thinking on what is real and true about the world so they may contribute to it in a meaningful way. Upon closer examination, however, to some extent these three conceptions are mutually incompatible, and not all are consistent with the core values of occupational therapy. These inconsistencies become even more striking when we consider the occupational therapy practitioner as the teacher and the clients of occupational therapy the students in the psychoeducation process.

Executive Approach

In this approach, the teacher is the "executor" of education, and therefore is responsible for determining what is to be taught, and then planning and delivering lesson content. In addition, the teacher acts as a manager of the students in the classroom or educational setting so that they proceed through prescribed learning activities in the way the teacher believes is most appropriate. In a similar way as executives in business firms do, the teacher in this model makes decisions about what people will do, when they will do it, how long it is likely to take, and what standard of performance determines whether to move to the next task or repeat the old one. Essentially, the executive teacher manages people and resources (Berliner, 1983).

The executive teacher, then, is far more than a content expert, though the content of learning is an important consideration. Emphasis in this approach is placed on the teacher's skill, such as being able to act friendly with the students in order to enlist their participation and maintain a cooperative relationship (Sedlak, Wheeler, Pullin & Cusik, 1986). Further emphasis is placed on the teacher's ability to maintain students engaged in the learning task through cues, corrective feedback and reinforcement (Waxman & Walberg, 1991). In other words, this conception of teaching emphasizes direct connection between what the teacher does and what the student learns–student learning is the product of the teacher's effectiveness in communicating or transmitting knowledge. In summary, the teacher assumes the responsibility for moving specific knowledge and skills from some outside source into the mind of the learner.

When comparing assumptions of the executive approach to occupational therapy values, certain conflicts arise. The teacher/therapist functions more like a manager of a production line, where students/clients are molded and shaped in order to reach a pre-determined standard. This standard is set by the teacher/therapist. In this approach, it is the student/clients who are involved in the process of education, while the teacher/therapist stays outside the process, directing it.

Psychoeducation programs designed and carried out within the framework of the executive approach emphasize a step-by-step curriculum. This curriculum is established by professional experts who, based on their expertise, have identified the knowledge clients need in order to be successful. Therefore, these programs often offer a lock-step progression of learning. For example, a program of this type might first introduce lectures by experts about various mental health disorders, followed by lectures about the usual treatment of such disorders. Some "practical" topics such as how to manage one's medication routine while at work, or even how to manage stress might be included in these programs. Worksheets to be completed by the client may be included as a method to maintain the client's attention. Two main characteristics are, however, that the teacher/expert takes responsibility for deciding which topics should be presented, and student/client adapts to the pre-established program which stresses attention to tasks and sequenced performance.

The executive approach is attractive to institutions and professionals because it provides a very efficient, clear, and straightforward means to move some specified knowledge into the mind of the client. The approach also makes it possible to make someone ultimately responsible for progress: the teacher/therapist. The teacher/therapist's effectiveness is measured by his/her ability to bring about learning by knowing precisely when and how to reinforce clients for behaviors that increasingly approximate the goals set for them.

The executive approach seems to disregard some fundamental elements of occupational therapy philosophy, such as the nature and interests of students/clients and their ability to influence their own health through occupation. Although psychoeducational experiences offered within this approach may include numerous purposeful activities or tasks, the evaluation of purposefulness lies within the teacher/therapist, not the student/client. Therefore, other core values of occupational therapy are ignored, including the student/client's choice to use his/her own capacities, to be self-directed, and to become self-actualized. Further, little consideration is given to each student/client's unique life context because the emphasis of the executive approach is on generic skills that all members of the class or group should master. This behaviorist, cause-and-effect conception of teaching and learning converts the client's therapeutic progress into a series of concrete and isolated events. The student/client must depend on the wisdom and knowledge of the teacher/therapist to not only sequence the events correctly, but to structure how these events are presented so that the client can produce the desired result. In this process, students/clients are not permitted to fully take charge of their own lives and actively realize their own particular meanings individually and as contributors to life in community. In fact, this approach relies on the maintenance of a relationship of dependence.

Therapist Approach

In contrast to the executive approach which emphasizes the content to be learned and the skills of the teacher, the therapist approach to teaching emphasizes the individual differences among students or learners. These differences are seen as impediments or facilitators of learning, and a core assumption is that who the learner is cannot be separated from what is learned and how it is learned (Fenstermacher & Soltis, 1998).

In the therapist approach, teaching is the process of guiding and assisting the learner to select the content and pursue the learning. Unlike the executive approach where teaching had mostly to do with preparing the content, the therapist teacher is more involved in preparing the learner for the tasks of choosing, working on, and evaluating what is learned. The purpose of teaching in the therapist approach is to enable the learner to become an authentic human being. This authenticity is cultivated by acquiring knowledge that is related to the quest for personal meaning and identity. Therefore, the learner's characteristics become the central focus of the teaching. The therapist teacher accepts responsibility for helping students make the choice to acquire specific knowledge, and then supports students as they advance their sense of self. In summary, in the therapist approach to teaching, the teacher is not one who imparts knowledge and skill to another, but one who helps another gain his own knowledge and skill. The teacher's task is to direct the learner inward so that the learner is then able to take responsibility for choices of actions that result from mastery of the content of learning (Rogers, 1964; Noddings & Shore, 1984).

Because the central concern in the therapist approach to teaching is the student/client's choice, this approach seems more akin to occupational therapy values. Rooted in humanist psychology from which occupational therapy has also derived much inspiration, the therapist approach to teaching stresses the uniqueness of individuals. Freedom, choice, personal growth, and the development of emotional and mental health are goals shared between the therapist approach to teaching and occupational therapy. The concern for the learner becoming an authentic human being finds particular echo in occupational therapy philosophy. Both perspectives view a self-actualized human being as one who possesses a balanced and integrated personality, and such traits as autonomy, creativeness, independence, altruism, and a healthy goal directedness (Maslow, 1962; Rogers, 1969; Fine, 1991; Kielhofner, 1997).

Given that the central concern of the therapist approach to teaching is the learner's individual growth, emphasis is placed on the learner's unique experience, or "experiential learning" (Rogers, 1969). The teacher or therapist does not impart knowledge. Instead, the teacher or therapist can only guide, suggest and encourage while the learner self-initiates and becomes fully and actively involved in the learning that has personal meaning to him or her. Thus, what is important is not what is taught, but rather, what is learned.

Psychoeducation provided from the therapist approach to teaching directs learners inward toward the self so that they can thereby reach outward and choose the content to be acquired and the actions to pursue. The most efficient way to provide this form of psychoeducation is likely to be individual, as each client uniquely seeks to find meaning through his or her actions. Any group instruction with specific objectives to learn a pre-determined content would necessarily negate the search for individuality and displace the client from the center of the therapeutic/learning process. Group instruction would not only homogenize the learners, it would emphasize the therapist teacher's control over the direction of learning.

The therapist approach to teaching is quite attractive to occupational therapy practitioners because it seems filled with dignity and hope for each human being. A concern which arises with this approach, however, is that its language of purpose, freedom, emotions, feelings, and subjective experience seem to center students/clients on themselves, incorporating caring for others only to the degree students/clients find it meaningful (Nodding, 1995). In this process, the common good, life in community, and responsibility toward contributing to a democratic society seem secondary.

Liberationist Approach

While the executive approach emphasizes teacher skill in transmitting specific knowledge and the therapist approach emphasizes the learner's ability to choose and acquire knowledge, a third approach can be identified that brings the knowledge, or content of learning itself, to the forefront. The aim of the liberationist approach to teaching is to free the student's mind from the limits of everyday experience, convention, and stereotype (Fenstermacher & Soltis, 1998). In contrast with the executive approach where knowledge is to be obtained and "had," or the therapist approach where knowledge is to be used for personal growth, in the liberationist approach knowledge is to be experienced critically (Peters, 1973; Bruner, 1987; Nodding, 1995 & 1999). A foundational belief of the liberationist approach is that knowledge inherently calls for particular actions and therefore, the teacher must teach by modeling such actions. In other words, in order to understand science, teachers and students must *do* science rather than simply learn *about* science; in order to understand literature, teachers and students must actively engage in creating literature; and so on. It is not the teacher as expert nor the student as personal meaning-seeker who determine what and how to learn. In the liberationist approach, it is the content or subject itself that that calls for specific ways of learning and acting.

The liberationist approach places great emphasis on the general manner in which teachers and learners face learning. Honesty, integrity, fair-mindedness, along with curiosity and judicious skepticism are to be developed at the same time as knowledge because learning comes about by *the way you learn* as well as from what you learn. The liberationist teacher must, therefore, teach these traits indirectly by modeling them as he or she learns alongside the students.

One thrust of liberationist thinking is related to the nature of knowledge itself, as explained above. Another thrust, however, is consideration of the social context in which learning occurs. This consideration is much broader than the group of students and teacher which surround each learner–it extends to the whole social world. Liberationism sees the whole world as a place of constant struggle and oppression in which people who have power assert themselves, and those who see themselves as inferior accept a fate of powerlessness. Liberationist thinkers argue that education is too often an instrument of an oppressive social system in which teachers have power and students do not, thus reproducing the broader context of society (Freire, 2000). The purpose of liberationist teaching is, then, to free the minds of students from the unconscious grip of oppressive ideas about their socioeconomic class, gender, race, or ethnicity because these ideas debilitate them and cut them off from a better life.

The two thrusts of liberationist teaching–that knowledge should be experienced, and that education should help one challenge oppression–come together in the notion of "critical consciousness" (Freire, 1974). In order to develop a critical consciousness, students and teachers must dialogue and collaborate, and together develop their images of a better, new reality. A critical consciousness arises when together teacher and students can step away from the unconscious acceptance of things the way they are and perceive the world critically in the midst of oppression. From this perspective, the ultimate aim of education is for students to liberate themselves to fully participate as equals in the classroom and in society (McLaren, 1989; Popkewitz, 1991; Noddings, 1999).

Liberationist thinking poses some interesting challenges to both the notion of psychoeducation and to occupational therapy practice. The development of a critical consciousness calls for not only the learning of various bodies of knowledge, but of the conceptual systems that underlie such knowledge (Freire, 2000). These conceptual systems are made of assumptions and values which should be questioned and examined critically. Therefore, from this perspective, psychoeducation (and the occupational therapy process itself) should begin with a questioning of the values which assume there even is a need for such education or treatment. Learning should not only involve the learner with the content and process of learning, but with the premises behind the need to learn (Mezirow, 2000). This can be an uncomfortable process, as it often will call into question the reasons that justify occupational therapy intervention.

Learning from the liberationist perspective does not end with an understanding of the values and assumptions that underlie knowledge. This approach calls for all participants (teacher and students alike) to critically examine their own values and assumptions because these play a significant role in the way in which each person perceives knowledge and the surrounding world. Only by understanding how these personal values and assumptions limit humans can the learner's mind be truly liberated. Of particular focus in the liberationist approach is the critical questioning of the values and assumptions learners hold that perpetuate a social system of oppression. In this approach, the development of self is only a step toward the development of the common good. The common good arises only when ". . . the person searches to be fully human by humanizing his fellow men and standing in solidarity together–a critical consciousness that knows one cannot be human as long as others are less than that" (Freire, 2000, p. 34). This solidarity can only be achieved through community.

From a liberationist perspective, psychoeducation would take on the form of dialogue in which both clients and occupational therapy practitioner openly discuss how their beliefs and actions contribute to their life in community, and to an oppressive or liberated society. The encounters between the occupational therapy practitioner and clients would be on an even plane, where the focus is not on the client's individual needs nor the practitioner's assessment of the client's need for development, but as "co-conspirators to humanize their life in community" (Mezirow, 2000, p. 26). The practitioner cannot be external to this process, but must be fully engaged with the client in the construction of meaning and of the future of society.

In this context, psychoeducation on stress management, for example, would include an examination of not only the physiology of stress and techniques to manage it, but also an examination of how each of us contributes to our own stress, each other's stress, and that of others. An essential discussion would include why we permit that cycle to continue. Further, an examination of how stress comes from and impacts our shared community in particular and society as a whole would be accompanied by an exploration of actions that we each can take, both as individuals and as a group, to effect a change not only in our own lives, but in society as a whole. Finally, that action should be undertaken together. This might lead us, for example, to make calls or write letters to government representatives, to participate in public protests, or to become involved in a community service program.

CONCLUSIONS

The three different ways of thinking about teaching presented here accomplish very different objectives. The executive approach emphasizes the transmission of information, the therapist approach emphasizes the search for personal meaning, and the liberationist approach emphasizes contribution to the common good. Psychoeducation undertaken from each of these approaches, then, also accomplishes different objectives. Given that occupational therapy practitioners often are involved in psychoeducational programs, the objectives of such programs must be evaluated in light of both the teaching approach and the philosophical values that should undergird all occupational therapy intervention.

Psychoeducation provided by occupational therapy practitioners from an executive approach appears to create the most obvious conflict of values. The practitioner stands in the center of this relationship, holding the power to decide what knowledge the client needs and how he/she will learn it. The emphasis on the therapeutic context rather than on the client's real life fragments the meaning such education may have, and stresses development of components of function rather than the integration of such components. Some may argue that many clients with mental conditions do not have the cognitive capacity to make sophisticated choices for themselves or others, and need first to develop abilities upon which to build choice. The result of this reasoning is occupational therapy intervention focused on developing components of function (for example, increasing attention or endurance). We know, however, that component-driven therapy is not effective (Trombly, 1995; Lin, Wu, Dengen & Coster, 1997). At any rate, the choice of psychoeducation would be inappropriate for clients with severe cognitive impairments because they would not be able to process cognitive information anyway. Because the executive approach de-emphasizes client agency, this form of psychoeducation cannot be considered authentic occupational therapy (Yerxa, 1966).

The therapist approach to teaching seems more compatible with occupational therapy values because, in contrast to the executive approach, it does emphasize client agency. However, because this approach is maintained through client uniqueness in making individual choices, the approach does not fully realize the occupational therapy value of contributing to the growth of social beings. Psychoeducation from this perspective would only address life in community if the client were to express such concern. Further, psychoeducation from this perspective would occur at the individual level because any group approach would homogenize people and de-emphasize their uniqueness. Therefore, the fullness of occupational therapy values may not be realized.

Finally, the liberationist approach to teaching offers a unique perspective to occupational therapy which challenges practitioner and client together to explore their relationship and critically examine the assumptions behind the notions of illness and need for therapy. The liberationist approach calls for the occupational therapy experience to be fully recognized as a real life experience in community, rather than preparation or training for life away from that relationship. Unlike the executive or therapist approaches explained above, the liberationist approach places the occupational therapy practitioner and the client as co-equals within the therapeutic learning process, so that as both learn together they form a learning community. In this sense, the occupational therapy process is one in which the client is brought into community, not only trained or prepared for it. The client's life or context cannot be seen as separate from the therapeutic one. Instead, we must understand how the therapeutic context fits into the wider life context of the client. Most importantly, we must critically consider whether the therapeutic experience is serving to actually liberate the client toward the fullness of life in society, or whether it is contributing to perpetuate in the client and in society the sense of being different and less than worthy to be included and seen as inherently equal.

Although the differences between these three approaches may at times seem subtle, they point to dramatically different outcomes of the therapeutic process. Ultimately, they bring into question the way in which we build a relationship with our clients and should guide how and why we use psychoeducation in the quest for providing authentic occupational therapy.

REFERENCES

American Occupational Therapy Association (1995-a). The philosophical base of occupational therapy. *American Journal of Occupational Therapy, 49*, 1026.

American Occupational Therapy Association (1995-b). Position paper: Occupation. *American Journal of Occupational Therapy, 49*, 1015-1018.

American Occupational Therapy Association (1993). Position paper: Purposeful activity. *American Journal of Occupational Therapy, 47*, 1981-1082.

Barris, R. (1985). Psychosocial occupational therapy education. *Mental Health Special Interest Section Newsletter, 7*, 4: 1-2.

Barter, J. (1984). Psychoeducation. In J. Talbott (Ed.) *The chronic mental patient: Five years later.* New York, NY: Grune & Stratton.

Bartlow, P. & Hartwig, C. (1989). Status of practice in mental health: Assessment and frames of reference. *Australian Occupational Therapy Journal, 36*, 180-192.

Berliner, D. (1983). The executive functions of teaching. *Instructor.* September: 29-39.

Bruner, J. (1987). *Actual minds, possible worlds.* Cambridge, MA: Harvard University Press.

Dickerson, A. (1996). Should choice be a component in occupational therapy assessment? *Occupational Therapy in Health Care, 10,* 3: 23-32.

Dixon, L. (1999). Providing services to families of persons with schizophrenia: Present and future. *Journal of Mental Health Policy and Economics, 2,* 3-8.

Dixon, L., Adams, C., & Lucksted, A. (2000). Update on family psychoeducation for schizophrenia. *Schizophrenia Bulletin, 26,* I: 5-20.

Englehardt, H. (1977). Defining occupational therapy: The meaning of therapy and the virtues of occupation. *American Journal of Occupational Therapy, 31,* 666-672.

Fenstermacher, G., & Soltis, J. (1998). *Approaches to teaching, 2nd ed.* New York, NY: Teacher's College Press.

Fine, S. (1991). Resilience and human adaptability: Who rises above adversity? The 1991 Eleanor Clarke Slagle lecture. *American Journal of Occupational Therapy, 45,* 493-403.

Freire, P. (2000). *Pedagogy of the oppressed (30th Anniversary Edition).* New York: Continuum Publications.

Freire, P. (1974). *Educating for critical consciousness.* New York: Continuum Publications.

Goldman, C. (1988). Toward a definition of psychoeducation. *Hospital and Community Psychiatry, 39,* 666-668.

Grady, A. P. (1995). Building inclusive community: A challenge for occupational therapy. The 1995 Eleanor Clarke Slagle Lecture. *American Journal of Occupational Therapy, 49,* 300-310.

Greenberg, L., Fine, S., Cohen, C., Larson, K., Michaelson-Baily, A., Rubinton, P., & Glick, I. (1988). In interdisciplinary psychoeducation program for schizophrenic patients and their families in an acute care setting. *Hospital and Community Psychiatry, 39,* 277-282.

Hayes, R. & Halford, W. (1993). Generalization of occupational therapy effects in psychiatric rehabilitation. *American Journal of Occupational Therapy, 47,* 161-167.

Henderson, A., Cermak, S., Coster, W., Murray, E., Trombly, C., & Tickle-Degnen, L. (1991). The issue is: Occupational science is multidimensional. *American Journal of Occupational Therapy, 45,* 370-372.

Kielhofner, G. (1995). *A model of human occupation: Theory and application. 2nd ed.* Baltimore, MD: Williams & Wilkins.

Kielhofner, G. (1997). *Conceptual foundations of occupational therapy, 2nd ed.* Philadelphia, PA: F.A. Davis.

Klasson, E. (1989). A model of the occupational therapist as case manager: Two case studies of chronic schizophrenic patients living in the community. *Occupational Therapy in Mental Health, 9,* 63-89.

Liberman, R., Wallace, C., Blackwell, G., Kopelowicz, A., Vaccaro, J., & Mints, J. (1998). Skills training versus psychosocial occupational therapy for persons with persistent schizophrenia. *American Journal of Psychiatry, 111,* 1087-1091.

Lin, K., Wu. C., Dengen, L. & Coster, W. (1997). Enhancing occupational performance through occupationally embedded exercise: A meta-analytic review. *Occupational Therapy Journal of Research, 17,* 25-47.

Lubin, H., Loris, M., Burt, J., & Johnson, D. (1998). Efficacy of psychoeducational group therapy in reducing symptoms of posttraumatic stress disorder among multiply traumatized women. *American Journal of Psychiatry, 155,* 1172-1177.

Maslow, A. (1962). *Toward a psychology of being.* New York: Van Nostrand.

McFarlane, W., Lukens, E., & Link, B. (1995). Multi-family groups and psycho-education in the treatment of schizophrenia. Multi-family groups and psychoeducation in the treatment of schizophrenia. *Archives of General Psychiatry, 52,* 679-687.

McLaren, P. (1989). *Life in schools: An introduction to critical pedagogy in the foundations of education.* New York: Longman.

Mezirow, J. (2000). *Learning as transformation: Critical perspectives on a theory in progress.* San Francisco, CA: Jossey-Bass.

Nelson, D. (1996). Therapeutic occupation: A definition. *American Journal of Occupational Therapy, 50,* 775-782.

Noddings, N. (1995). *Philosophy of education.* New York: Westview Press.

Noddings, N. (1999). *Justice and caring: The search for common ground in education.* New York: Teachers College Press.

Noddings, N. & Shore, P. (1984). *Awakening the inner eye: Intuition in education.* New York: Teachers College Press.

Peters, R. (1973). *The philosophy of education.* London: Oxford University Press.

Pollio, D., North, C., & Foster (1998). Content and curriculum in psychoeducation groups for families of persons with severe mental illness. *Psychiatric Services, 49,* 816-822.

Popkewitz, T. (1991). *A political sociology of educational reform: Power/knowledge in teaching, teacher education, and research.* New York: Teachers College Press.

Reilly, M. (1966). A psychiatric occupational therapy program as a teaching model. *American Journal of Occupational Therapy, 20,* 60-67.

Rogers, C. (1969). *Freedom to learn.* Columbus, OH: Charles E. Merrill.

Sedlak, M., Wheeler, D., Pullin, C. & Cusik, A. (1986). *Selling students short: Classroom bargains and academic reform in the American high school.* New York: Teacher's College Press.

Solomon, P. (1996). Moving from psychoeducation to education of families of adults with serious mental illness. *Psychiatric Services, 47,* 1364-1370.

Spencer, J., Glick, I., Haas, G., Claekin, J., Lewis, A., Peyser, J., DeMane, N., Good-Ellis, M., Harris, E., & Lestelle, V. (1988). A randomized clinical trial of in-patient family intervention: Effects at 6-month and 18-month follow-ups. *American Journal of Psychiatry, 145,* 1115-1121.

Trombly, C. (1995). Occupation: Purposefulness and meaningfulness as therapeutic mechanisms: The 1995 Eleanor Clarke Slagle Lecture. *American Journal of Occupational Therapy, 49,* 960-972.

Wallace, C., Liberman, R., MacKain, S., Blackwell, G., & Eckman, T. (1992). Effectiveness and replicability of modules for teaching social and instrumental skills to the severely mentally ill. *American Journal of Psychiatry, 149,* 654-658.

Waxman, H. & Walberg, H. (1991). *Effective teaching: Current research.* Berkeley, CA: McCutchan.

Yerxa, E. (1967). Authentic occupational therapy: The 1966 Eleanor Clarke Slagle Lecture. *American Journal of Occupational Therapy, 21,* 1-9.

Yerxa, E., Clark, F., Frank, G., Jackson, J., Parham, D., Pierce, D., Stein, C., & Zemke, R. (1990). An introduction to occupational science: A foundation for occupational therapy in the 21st century. *Occupational Therapy in Health Care, 4,* 2, 1-17.

PART THREE:
APPLICATION
OF RECOVERY PRINCIPLES

Recovery and Occupational Therapy in the Community Mental Health Setting

Jason L. Wollenberg, OTR

SUMMARY. The purpose of this essay is to describe how occupational therapy operates in a community mental health setting focused on recovery and wellness, from the perspective of a first year occupational therapist. The philosophy of recovery and wellness coincides with a philosophy of intervention that is consumer centered and consumer driven. Occupational therapy began in this setting through a fieldwork relationship between the mental health center and an occupational therapy education program. As the first occupational therapist hired as staff, the author developed an occupational therapy program that corresponds to the principles of recovery. The relationship between occupational therapy and recovery and wellness is described by

Jason L. Wollenberg is Community Integration Specialist, Wyandot Center for Community Behavioral Healthcare, Inc, 1223 Meadowlark Lane, Kansas City, KS 66102.

[Haworth co-indexing entry note]: "Recovery and Occupational Therapy in the Community Mental Health Setting." Wollenberg, Jason L. Co-published simultaneously in *Occupational Therapy in Mental Health* (The Haworth Press, Inc.) Vol. 17, No. 3/4, 2001, pp. 97-114; and: *Recovery and Wellness: Models of Hope and Empowerment for People with Mental Illness* (ed: Catana Brown) The Haworth Press, Inc., 2001, pp. 97-114. Single or multiple copies of this article are available for a fee from The Haworth Document Delivery Service [1-800-HAWORTH, 9:00 a.m. - 5:00 p.m. (EST). E-mail address: getinfo@haworthpressinc.com].

97

outlining the occupational therapy process. From referral to discontinuation, the unique aspects of practicing in a recovery and wellness setting are depicted. Finally, a case study illustrates one example of the relationship between recovery and occupational therapy in the community mental health setting. *[Article copies available for a fee from The Haworth Document Delivery Service: 1-800-HAWORTH. E-mail address: <getinfo@haworthpressinc.com> Website: <http://www.HaworthPress.com> © 2001 by The Haworth Press, Inc. All rights reserved.]*

KEYWORDS. Recovery, occupational therapy, community, mental health, process

BACKGROUND

As a recent occupational therapy graduate, I was faced with the unique opportunity to become the first occupational therapist on staff at a metropolitan community mental health center. During my tenure as a student, I had the privilege of completing a Level II fieldwork placement at this same facility. The occupational therapy education program at the University of Kansas Medical Center had built a fieldwork relationship with the mental health center's community support services over several years. Students completed their fieldwork education under the supervision of a faculty member and began to build an occupational therapy program where one had not existed before. I happened to be one of the students in a long line that created and refined the role of occupational therapy in this setting, and developed the procedures to deliver our service. The mental health center was open to the unique services we were able to provide and expressed this openness by creating a staff position for an occupational therapist. This new position provided a wonderful opportunity for the expansion of occupational therapy services in the community mental health setting. I was excited to be given the responsibility of building on the foundation created by fieldwork students over the previous years.

PARTNERSHIP IN RECOVERY

The relationship between occupational therapy and the mental health center grew primarily because of a shared philosophy of practice. All of the services provided at the mental health center emphasize the principle of recovery. This principle is a shift away from the treatment model that was aimed at merely stabilizing consumers with mental illnesses. In the former model, if the person was not hospitalized and he or she was relatively symptom free, he or she would be considered stable. Because the consumer was stable, there would be less need for services unless there was a risk for hospitalization or an exacerbation of symptoms. This philosophy does not address the scope of the issues faced by persons who experience mental illness. Dreams and ambition do not die with the diagnosis of a mental illness, yet previous treatment only provided help with an attempt to reduce symptoms and to keep the individual out of the hospital. The recovery model provides help to consumers as they move to achieve their personal goals and ambitions in life. The community mental health center provides services that foster this recovery. For example, classes are provided in which consumers can bring their family members or significant others to learn about mental illness in the framework of recovery. Other services include groups that provide skills for self-advocacy, political awareness, and fighting stigma.

There is also a community atmosphere in which consumers have role models in other consumers who are on the recovery journey. The atmosphere and focus on recovery creates an environment in the organization that is positive and exciting. Occupational therapy fits very well into the array of services that consumers can access to help them in their personal recovery journey. We are able to teach skills, modify tasks, or adapt the environment to help the consumer achieve their goals to the fullest potential. The agency recognized the extremely positive benefits of occupational therapy to provide these unique and otherwise unavailable services to consumers in the recovery model.

The focus on recovery and wellness produces an environment that allows the service recipient, or consumer, to be the primary decision-maker and stakeholder in the services he or she receives. For many, deciding on the services one receives seems to be common sense. However, the history of treatment in mental health paints a very different picture that conflicts with this line of thinking. For years, the only option for treatment was to be admitted to a psychiatric ward where the individual had very little say in the services that he or she was to receive. The recovery and wellness focus of the community mental health setting has changed the focus and even the semantics of treatment in which the patient/client is now considered a consumer of mental health services. This change in semantics reflects an important shift in how services are provided for individuals who want and need mental health services. Because of this shift, the consumer is now the most important person involved in intervention and service planning. The manner in which service planning takes place at this specific community mental health setting reflects the prominent role of the consumer in a recovery and wellness model.

The consumer works on a personal service plan with his or her case manager to set goals and devise a plan to reach these goals. The long-term goals, indicated on each consumer's individual service plan, are set by the consumer and are in their own language. Any service rendered in this system must relate directly to a goal that has been identified by the consumer. Because the consumer sets his or her own goals, the content of the goal often relates to practical daily life. For example, several consumers have goals that relate to maintaining or obtaining independent living status. These goals provide a tremendous opportunity for occupational therapy to provide services to the consumer and assist in their progress toward their recovery goals. After setting goals and revising them periodically, the consumer continues to have the final say in the services that he or she receives to address these goals.

The community mental health center offers case management, vocational rehabilitation, homeless crisis and support, medicine clinic, psychosocial rehabilitation, a peer wellness and support program, and now occupational therapy. Consumers are educated and made aware of the services available, and may be referred to one or more of the programs previously outlined. However, it is ultimately the consumer's decision to utilize the services that can help them achieve their goals. For example, an individual might have goals to maintain their independent living status and increase their socialization. This person currently is having trouble with keeping her apartment clean and she tends to become isolated and bored at home. The case manager would present the options available and help the person select the appropriate services. For example, the case manager could suggest that the consumer attend psychosocial rehabilitation groups to help increase her socialization activities and reduce boredom. It may also be suggested that a referral be made to occupational therapy to help develop a system to keep her apartment clean. Finally, a referral to the vocational team to start job searches or pre-vocational training may be suggested.

In this very common situation, the consumer may elect to begin participating in social and recreational groups and to begin working with occupational therapy on her home maintenance. However, she may decide that she is not ready to start thinking about work at this point in her recovery, but would like to keep the option open for the future. This example illustrates the manner in which recovery allows the consumer to set his or her own priorities for receiving services. Furthermore, it demonstrates that this system provides a unique opportunity and niche for occupational therapy to serve as a positive support for mental health consumers in the recovery process.

PURPOSE

The purpose of this essay is to describe how occupational therapy operates in a community mental health setting focused on recovery and wellness, from the perspective of a first year occupational therapist. The recovery model has a tremendous impact on every aspect of the occupational therapy process (American Occupational Therapy Association, 2000). For this reason, I have elected to describe each step of the occupational therapy process and the manner in which the recovery model has guided the development and implementation of the procedures in providing occupational therapy services. It is not intended to be a logistical outline of the occupational therapy process, but a framework to provide a comprehensive picture of occupational therapy and its relationship to recovery in a community mental health setting. There are a wide variety of issues and needs that occupational therapy addresses in this setting. Although it is a mental health setting, many physical disability issues arise. The wellness and recovery model guides us to see the person from a holistic perspective and to provide interventions in kind.

Physical disability issues such as diabetes, arthritis, incontinence, stroke recovery, or various broken bones are at times the primary reason a consumer is referred to occupational therapy. However, because of the individual's mental health needs, the consumer has unique challenges to manage or recover from due to his or her physical issue. In fact, he or she may need more assistance with the stress and life changes that have been created by the physical problem than help with the physical problem itself. Throughout the occupational process, it is important to understand the relationship and balance between physical and mental wellness. From referral to discontinuation or transition, the concept of recovery has guided the manner in which we have developed and practiced occupational therapy.

STEP 1: REFERRAL

The first step in the occupational therapy process also provided the first challenge in providing services in this community mental health setting. To provide occupational therapy, we needed a method for consumers to be referred to our services. For consumers to be referred to our services, we needed to educate other professionals and consumers about occupational therapy and the types of assessments and interventions we can provide. The previous years of an active fieldwork program allowed the staff and consumers at the mental health center to become familiar with the skills and services available with occupational therapists. However, each group of fieldwork students faced the need to expand and refine what the previous group established. This expansion and refinement took time and required us to market the services again to staff and consumers. This marketing took the form of meeting with case managers, consumers, and other staff to educate them on the scope of occupational therapy in this setting. Marketing also involved developing a useful, understandable, and comprehensive referral form to reinforce the areas in which individual consumers could benefit from occupational therapy service.

The recovery model has now become an essential guiding principle for marketing our service as well as guidance for the framework of the referral form. We currently market occupational therapy as an additional tool available to the consumer for their recovery journey. The referral form reflects this focus by providing a scale to identify the consumer's stage in recovery (Figure 1). By integrating recovery into the referral process, occupational therapy has become an integrated piece of the overall recovery model.

What does the referral process look like in this setting with the recovery model? Not only do we accept referrals from case managers and other staff, but we also accept self-referrals from the consumers. The recovery model emphasizes the personal investment and desire to better oneself. Therefore, it is essential that self-referral be an option to allow occupational therapy to support the individual's recovery process. In practice, the majority of the referrals come from case managers. Because case managers usually have the closest professional relationship with the consumer, it is important for occupational therapy to educate and inform the case management teams on the services we can provide. Then the case manager has the knowledge to refer the consumer to our service to support the individual's recovery. The referral form provides us with information such as: a name, a broad treatment goal, an idea of

FIGURE 1. This Is the Occupational Therapy Referral Form Currently Used in This Community Mental Health Setting. In Addition to Basic Background Information and Areas for Specific Skill Development, It Includes a Scale to Identify the Consumer's Stage in Recovery

Occupational Therapy Referral

Consumer Name: _____ ID Number: _____
Address: _____ Telephone: _____

Case Manager: _____

Reason for Referral: _____
_____
_____

Please provide a goal from the Individual Service Plan that corresponds to the requested service.
Domain: _____
Goal: _____
_____

At What Stage of Recovery Do You See This Consumer?

Overcoming Stuckness	Returning to Basic Functioning	Discovering Self-empowerment	Learning and Self-redefinition	Improving Quality of Life
-Acknowledging and accepting illness -Desire and motivation to change -Finding/having source of hope/ inspiration	-Taking care of basic needs: eating, hygiene, basic physical health -Being active: exercising, leisure activities -Connecting with others	-Taking responsibility for own recovery -Taking responsibility for behaviors -Determined and hard working -Courage to challenge self and take risks	-Recapturing parts of old self and discovering new aspects of self -Learning there is more to self than illness	-Striving to attain overall sense of well-being -Striving for ideals often associated with stable mental health -Serving as a recovery role model for others

Areas of Specific Skill Development (please check all that apply)

Self-Management
☐ Grooming/Hygiene (bathing, dressing, oral hygiene, etc...)
☐ Health Maintenance (nutrition, fitness socialization, etc...)
☐ Life/Stress Management
☐ Personal and Community Safety
☐ Community Mobility
☐ Other _____

Household Management
☐ Cleaning
☐ Laundry
☐ Shopping
☐ Money Management
☐ Child/Elder Care
☐ Meal Preparation
☐ Other _____

Community Participation
☐ Interpersonal Relationships (conflict resolution, communication)
☐ Vocational Participation
☐ Educational Preparation
☐ Leisure/Recreational Participation
☐ Community Responsibility
☐ Other _____

Additional comments: _____
_____
_____

Referred by: _____ Date: _____

the consumer's stage of recovery, and specific areas for desired skill development. After obtaining the referral, the next step in the occupational therapy process is screening, which is also influenced by the recovery model.

STEP 2: SCREENING

The screening process insures that the occupational therapist will have enough information to select proper and useful assessments to evaluate the consumer. It can also be used to determine whether occupational therapy is appropriate, or if a referral to another professional is needed. The most basic and familiar part of the process is the chart review. It is useful to gather diagnostic and historical treatment information to get a better sense of the issues that may be involved. This chart review also provides details on what the individual has been working on with other members of the treatment team. To help the consumer progress toward his or her recovery goals, this knowledge helps the occupational therapist understand where an intervention would be most beneficial. However, reviewing the chart alone falls far short of the necessary actions for the screening process in this setting. There are two persons to interview before any formal evaluation begins. The case manager has a unique insight into the issues that warranted a referral to occupational therapy. Many times the case manager will elaborate in greater detail about the issues in a face-to-face discussion than they indicated on the referral. They also have wonderful information about the best way to contact the consumer, communication styles, and other useful logistics. The case manager will continue to be a useful resource and a close contact during the time that occupational therapy is working with the consumer.

The second and most important person to interview before formal evaluation is the consumer. This aspect of the screening process is essential in the recovery model. The consumer needs to actually want help with the issues that were indicated in the referral and be willing to work with occupational therapy to make progress toward his or her recovery goals. Given that the consumer is invested in working on the issue, this is also the time to ascertain their expectations and goals for intervention from occupational therapy. At this point if the consumer or case manager elaborates on the issue and it is outside the scope of occupational therapy, a referral to another professional and/or education on other sources of assistance are provided. It is also possible, and not uncommon, that the consumer does not want or is not invested in receiving service from occupational therapy. As part of the recovery model, this is the consumer's decision to make. An intervention would not likely be successful with an individual who was not interested in working on the issue. However, the recovery model also empowers those consumers interested in change to be the authors of their own recovery. This screening interview allows the consumer to express the direction and purpose of the occupational therapy intervention.

STEP 3: EVALUATION

The knowledge gained from the referral and screening process allows the occupational therapist to select an appropriate evaluation method. The specific method that is selected varies greatly depending on the consumer and his or her situation. Without undergoing the steps in the screening process, it would be difficult to select relevant assessments appropriate for the particular consumer. However, in this setting, the therapist has taken the steps to interview the consumer and case manager before the evaluation, which eases the selection of appropriate and useful assessments. Because the issues generally raised for OT intervention involve functional daily life issues, the evaluation process almost always includes interviews and structured observations with the consumer. The observations and interview are generally conducted in the natural setting that the consumer normally uses. For example, a consumer who has been referred for meal preparation skills would be observed preparing a meal in their own home. Formal assessments are also used in adjunct, when necessary, to help evaluate the scope of the issues the consumer wishes to address. The recovery model is evident in this process through the selection of assessments that help provide information specific to the consumer's goals for recovery. It is also important that the logistics and procedures involved in the assessment are appropriate in respect to the individual's stage of recovery.

An example of the evaluation process in this setting begins with a consumer who was referred because of hygiene concerns. In the process of screening and the initial interview, the consumer related that he did not feel his hygiene was as much of an issue as others thought it was. However, he wanted to increase his socialization and specifically, he wanted to get a girlfriend. It hurt his feelings as well as his chance to achieve his goals when he heard others commenting on his poor hygiene. For this reason, he decided to explore the issue with occupational therapy, even though he did not think the problem was that bad.

The first aspect of the evaluation process was this first interview where observation determined through both senses of sight and smell that hygiene was indeed an issue that needed attention. It also raised suspicion that his sensory processing was affecting how he perceived his hygiene. As an adjunct to the observation and interview, the Adult Sensory Profile (Brown, Tollefson, Dunn, Cromwell, and Filion, 2001) was used to explore his sensory processing and guide future intervention planning. The results of this more formal assessment revealed that the consumer had low sensory registration. In other words, he required more sensory input than normal to recognize sensory triggers such as odors. These findings, in addition to observations and interviews, provided useful information to support the intervention planning process.

The consumer was concerned with the comments of others about his hygiene, but he did not fully understand the basis of their comments. This evaluation process supported his recovery journey by providing him an explanation of why he was not sensing his hygiene as others were. This shared knowledge between the occupational therapist and the consumer provided a strong foundation for working together to find a solution to the barriers that were keeping him from his goals.

STEP 4: INTERVENTION PLANNING

Intervention planning is a collaborative effort between the occupational therapist and the consumer. This collaboration reflects the manner in which recovery impacts this step in the occupational therapy process. Recovery also empowers each individual to focus on their hopes and dreams in life, not just on reducing symptoms or eliminating problems. Therefore, a large part of intervention planning is used to encourage the consumer to focus on the goals he or she has in life. In turn, we collaborate to determine the barriers that are keeping them from achieving those goals. Following this discussion and the evaluation process, the knowledge of the barriers to accomplishing the consumer's goals can be used to make plans for interventions that will help the individual overcome the barriers. One of the primary tasks in this stage is to set the long- and short-term goals for occupational therapy intervention. If the occupational therapist were to set these goals for the consumer, that action would be in conflict with the principles of the recovery model. In recovery, the consumer should be involved in as much of the intervention process as possible, especially when setting goals. The occupational therapist works with the individual to articulate the long-term goals for intervention, as well as the short-term objectives to accomplish those goals. The consumer provides his or her insight on the areas in which they have a personal investment to improve. The occupational therapist brings clinical judgement and reasoning to help the consumer set reasonable and attainable goals.

The other aspect of intervention planning is the creation of a roadmap of interventions that will help the consumer achieve the short-term objectives and in turn the long-term goal. This requires the clinical reasoning of the therapist to use the information attained from screening and evaluation to select relevant interventions. However, the consumer may not approve of a specific intervention in the plan for a variety of reasons. They may have experienced the same intervention in the past with little success or may be uncomfortable with its physical or mental requirements. Consumers are urged not to eliminate challenge from their treatment, but in recovery it is up to the individual to decide the amount of challenge he or she wishes to experience. The consumer makes the ultimate decision on the goals and interventions that are written into the intervention plan.

Previous models in mental health resembled the medical model, in which the professional or expert prescribed the intervention that he or she felt would be of greatest benefit for the individual. Not only does the medical model discount the unique life experience of each individual; it is not effective in establishing a collaborative and productive relationship with the consumer. When the occupational therapist works with the consumer in a cooperative manner, any doubts about relinquishing total decision making to the consumer quickly subside. The consumer can provide input on his or her motivations, any successful or unsuccessful strategies used to address problems in the past, and insight into the areas that he or she would like to address in the future. The empowerment of the consumer empowers the occupational therapist to use his or her clinical reasoning to develop effective interventions. The collaboration exhibited in the intervention planning process solidifies the foundation for occupational therapy to be a very beneficial resource in the consumer's recovery.

STEP 5: INTERVENTION

The preparation from the screening, assessment, and intervention planning processes allows the occupational therapist to provide interventions to meet the established goals. The preceding steps in the occupational therapy process have been completed with recovery and wellness as a guiding principle, so the actual interventions that emerge will support the consumer's occupational performance and recovery. The natural environment of the consumer is important as interventions are provided. The knowledge and skill that is gained during the intervention will better carry over to life when it is gained in the natural setting. Therefore, our interventions typically take place in the consumer's home, at a local grocery store, or other community settings.

There are also situations in which community resources are utilized to provide the education or skill building that the consumer needs. For example, a consumer with a recent diagnosis of diabetes was not very knowledgeable about the disease or the care and prevention steps he needed to take. The occupational therapist and the consumer in this case found a community diabetes support group that the individual was interested in attending. The therapist was then able to support and assist the consumer in managing and applying the information he received from the support group. This community resource became an important component of the intervention and the intervention plan.

In addition to the natural environment and use of community resources, family members and significant others sometimes play an important role in the consumer's recovery. Through collaboration with the consumer in this process, it becomes apparent whether a spouse, parent, child, or friend is important to the intervention process. However, if the consumer does not want a family member or significant other involved, that wish is always respected.

There is an interesting parallel that seems to exist between recovery and occupational performance. In any setting, an improvement in occupational performance is the desired outcome for occupational therapy. In fact, the term recovery is not limited to the mental health setting. For example, when an individual is undergoing rehabilitation from hip surgery, we could also say that this individual is recovering from the surgery. This person would benefit from occupational therapy because their occupational performance has been reduced. The purpose and direction of occupational therapy intervention is focused on helping the person regain their occupational performance in daily living tasks, work or productive activities, and/or leisure or recreation. As the individual participates in therapy, the performance in these areas increases and one could say that they are undergoing *recovery* from the injury.

The consumer of mental health services can also experience reductions in occupational performance. Once again, the purpose and direction of occupational therapy intervention is aimed at helping the individual increase his or her participation and satisfaction with occupational performance in daily living tasks, work or productive activities, and/or leisure or recreation. The consumer participates in daily life. Like the patient who had hip surgery, increased participation and satisfaction with occupational performance for the consumer is synonymous with progress in recovery. This parallel between recovery and occupational performance reinforces the fit of occupational therapy within the recovery model.

Implementation of the intervention plan allows the consumer to improve his or her occupational performance as previously set goals are reached. However, implementing interventions often requires flexibility with the original plan. The consumer may not feel challenged by the intervention, or it may be too challenging. In this situation, the activity may need to be graded, respectively, to be more or less of a challenge. The consumer could also find that the planned intervention was not fulfilling or stimulating enough to keep them invested in the activity. This situation may require selection of an entirely different approach to help the consumer achieve his or her goals. These situations, and any others that cause the intervention to be ineffectual, are evaluated to determine what type of modification needs to be made to the interventions.

STEP 6: REEVALUATION

The consumer is also reevaluated to determine the progress that has been made toward his or her goals. With this process, the occupational therapist and the consumer can determine what, if any, changes need to be made to the intervention plan. Once again, the recovery model encourages the consumer to be an active participant in the provision of his or her own services. The partnership of the occupational therapist and the consumer creates an environment of shared responsibility and effort. Rather than having a passive role in the intervention process, the consumer is empowered to be actively involved in the process. Consequently, the empowered consumer enhances the ability of the occupational therapist to provide services more efficiently and effectively. The focus on teamwork provides a positive environment for the therapist as well as the consumer. With this focus, the consumer and the practitioner become a team that is working together to achieve the consumer's goals for recovery.

STEP 7: DISCONTINUATION/TRANSITION

The eventual destination of the occupational therapy process is the discontinuation of service or transition to further services. There are several ways to reach this step in the process as it operates in this recovery-focused setting. Again, the consumer is the primary decision-maker as to whether to discontinue occupational therapy services. This decision may come at any point in the occupational therapy process. For example, some consumers decide that they do not want occupational therapy services during the initial screening interview. This situation occurs when the referral source feels that the consumer would benefit from occupational therapy, but the consumer feels that he or she is not at a place in their recovery to take those steps. An individual who has been informed about occupational therapy, but is not ready to utilize it, will not benefit from services that are not desired at that particular point in time. It is best to discontinue the service and leave the door open for the individual to address the needs when he or she feels ready to do so.

A more gratifying example of the need to discontinue service occurs when all the goals have been accomplished and the consumer is satisfied with his or her progress. The occupational therapist ensures that proper supports are in place to help the consumer maintain the progress that was made. In this situation, the issue that prompted the referral has been resolved. There have also been situations when the occupational therapist who is working with a consumer must leave the agency due to the completion of a fieldwork, vacation, or possibly a job change. When the consumer is still receiving services from occupational therapy, the services are transitioned to another occupational therapist.

Finally, the occupational therapist may determine that the individual's needs are not within the scope of occupational therapy. Then the occupational therapist can help the consumer to identify other resources available that could help resolve the issue. With the agreement of the individual, the therapist should make a referral to a professional with the expertise to address the issue. The completion of the occupational therapy process provides another illustration of how consumer empowerment through recovery influences the delivery of occupational therapy services. The following case study represents the occupational therapy process and its relationship to recovery and wellness, following the steps as they have been outlined above.

CASE STUDY–KAREN

Karen was referred to occupational therapy by her case manager. This particular case manager is very familiar with occupational therapy and has made several referrals in the past. As a long time case manager with the agency, she had experienced several groups of occupational therapy students and their educational promotions of occupational therapy. The case manager indicated the following reason for referring Karen: "Moving out of nursing home into apartment, had stroke, partially blind. Really forgetful, doesn't know what skills she has retained." She also checked *Cleaning, Laundry,* and *Meal Preparation* as areas for specific skill development. The case manager indicated Karen was in a stage of recovery in which she was beginning to discover self-empowerment. Finally, the overarching consumer goal that was listed on the referral was "Live independently." The information gained from this referral provided direction for further steps in the process.

The screening process allowed the occupational therapist to gather background information from Karen's chart and her case manager. These sources indicated that the primary issues at the time were related to her poor eyesight and impaired memory due to a stroke which occurred two years previously, diabetes, and other health problems. The consumer indicated that these barriers were interfering with her ability to live independently and to feel safe performing daily tasks such as cleaning, laundry, and making meals. Karen was especially interested in increasing her abilities in the kitchen and indicated displeasure in her inability to read due to low vision.

Following the screening step in the occupational therapy process, the therapist determined that a home evaluation and observation of Karen during meal planning would be the most appropriate assessment. The therapist set up a time to meet with Karen in her apartment to conduct the evaluation. During the evaluation, the occupational therapist noticed that the lighting in the kitchen was very dim and that Karen had an extremely difficult time reading the small numbers on the oven dials. The therapist also observed that the books Karen wanted to read were printed with standard size type that was too small for her to read without aid. These observations led the therapist into a discussion with the consumer about planning interventions that would assist her in these areas.

The occupational therapist suggested increasing the lighting in the kitchen and the use of puffy paint on the oven dials as a visual and tactile cueing strategy. Karen agreed that these plans would help in the kitchen. For reading, the therapist suggested options such as large print books, a magnifying glass, reading glasses, or audio books. Once again, Karen was open to these suggestions, except for the audio books. She had tried these in the past and was unable to retain the information by hearing it. This made audio books very undesirable because she could not remember earlier portions of the book that gave meaning to the entire story. Finally, the occupational therapist and Karen agreed on developing a large calendar as a memory aid. The knowledge that Karen brought to the intervention planning process was extremely valuable and steered the intervention away from a strategy that she knew did not work for her.

The collaboration of the therapist and consumer in the planning process set the tone for partnership and progress in the intervention stage. As the occupational therapist worked with Karen on the interventions that they had planned together, she had the opportunity to constantly monitor the progress and reevaluate the consumer's skills. When she developed skills in one area, they were able to plan interventions and collaborate on another area that needed improvement.

The first intervention that made a tremendous impact for Karen's functioning was the purchase of a magnifying glass. It was an adaptation that made the tasks of reading both books and oven dials much more manageable. Karen was very pleased with the results, which motivated her to work toward other goals. However, one problem that Karen was having was difficulty remembering her appointments not only with occupational therapy, but her case manager, other professionals, and her friends and relatives. The next step in the intervention process involved the development of a large calendar that would be functional for Karen, improve her orientation, and provide cues for remembering appointments and engagements. Once again, the collaboration was crucial to empower Karen in her recovery and to create an intervention that was likely to succeed. The calendar provided the necessary cues that Karen needed to remember the tasks, activities, and appointments each day. Other professionals and her relatives began writing appointments, activities, and other information on her calendar, which made it even more functional and useful to the consumer. The success of the interventions and the willingness of the therapist to collaborate with Karen encouraged her to press on with other goals.

As the therapeutic relationship grew, the skills that Karen acquired grew as well. She began to venture into other areas for skill development as well as expand the skills she had recently regained. Karen indicated to the occupational therapist that she wanted to work on laundering her clothes in the laundry room of her apartment. She had been struggling with the process and was getting overwhelmed to the point that she neglected to do her laundry. Once again, through collaboration, the therapist and Karen developed strategies that allowed her to become more independent with her laundry. They used strategies such as measuring the proper amount of detergent into a plastic bag to take to the laundry room instead of the entire box, sorting the clothes in the apartment before going to the laundry room, and using magnets to place on the washers and dryers she was using to help her remember which machines held her clothes.

As Karen's confidence in her abilities grew, she began to express interest in more complex cooking tasks. She felt comfortable baking a cake independently with some assistance in the set up. The occupational therapist assisted her in getting the supplies and ingredients out and reviewed oven operation and safety before leaving her with the task. Karen proudly reported to the therapist that she completed this task and was extremely pleased with the results. The occupational therapist reflected that Karen was making progress by not only expressing and following through with interests, but also feeling more confident in her ability to perform activities. Karen and the therapist built on this confidence by exploring more cooking opportunities and adapting recipes to meet her physical and nutritional needs.

At the same time, Karen was becoming more confident in social situations and expressed more interest in groups provided by the community mental health center and her apartment. The confidence gained from successes related to cooking and cleaning seemed to carry over to other areas of her life. The fact that Karen was the primary decision maker in the therapeutic relationship could only have strengthened her feelings of empowerment and confidence.

Because the therapist working with Karen was a Level II Fieldwork student, a transition of services to another therapist would be needed. After meeting for the final time, Karen and the therapist collectively decided to transition her to the next occupational therapist to continue working on her goals. In the transition referral the occupational therapist gave a brief synopsis of the focus of therapeutic interventions during her time working with Karen. She also provided recommendations for future occupational therapy focus. Because of Karen's increasing confidence, she recommended that the new therapist encourage an increase in social activities and provide the necessary supports for success. She also indicated areas that Karen was interested in exploring with future occupational therapy services. Karen was interested in assistance with developing a grocery list for her special diabetic dietary needs as well as becoming more involved in social and leisure activities in the community.

Next, the occupational therapist recommended the continued encouragement to use the calendar and the magnifying glass, which required some prompting on several occasions. Finally, she recommended that the future therapist empower and challenge Karen to take part in activities even when she lacks confidence in her ability to do so. Karen often succeeded in areas where she lacked confidence when she was provided encouragement and support. This case study illustrates the impact that the focus on recovery and wellness has on the occupational therapy process. The collaborative therapeutic relationship demonstrated in this example was very beneficial for the consumer. The teamwork between the therapist and the consumer created an environment that fostered progress and success.

CONCLUSION

The unique opportunity to start my career in a community mental health setting, as the first occupational therapist on staff, has been rewarding and educational. It has also been a unique experience because this setting has adopted the relatively new concept of recovery and wellness as the model of service delivery. I have found that occupational therapy fits into this system beautifully. Through the development and implementation of an occupational therapy program, I have witnessed the role for occupational therapy develop harmoniously with the recovery model. It addresses needs for consumers that are unique from the needs addressed by other professions in the setting. As consumers of mental health services embark on personal journeys of recovery, occupational therapy can provide the extra support that may be needed to reach the destination.

REFERENCES

American Occupational Therapy Association. (2000). *The Reference Manual of the Official Documents of the American Occupational Therapy Association, Inc.* Bethesda, MD: Author.

Brown, C., Tollefson, N., Dunn, W., Cromwell, R., & Filion, D. (2001). Adult Sensory Profile: Measuring patterns of sensory processing. *American Journal of Occupational Therapy, 55*, 75-82.

What Is the Best Environment for Me?
A Sensory Processing Perspective

Catana Brown, PhD, OTR, FAOTA

SUMMARY. This paper describes the process of evaluating and designing interventions for sensory processing preferences using the *Adult Sensory Profile*. The measure is theoretically based on Dunn's Model of Sensory Processing (1997) which describes the intersection of neurological threshold and behavioral responses resulting in the following four quadrants: sensory sensitivity, sensation avoiding, low registration and sensation seeking. The compatibility of this model and recovery is discussed along with specific strategies for matching environments and sensory processing preferences. *[Article copies available for a fee from The Haworth Document Delivery Service: 1-800-HAWORTH. E-mail address: <getinfo@haworthpressinc.com> Website: <http://www.HaworthPress.com> © 2001 by The Haworth Press, Inc. All rights reserved.]*

KEYWORDS. Neurological threshold, sensation, behavioral response, environment

INTRODUCTION

If asked to describe your sensory processing preferences, most people would not know what to say. However, every minute of every day,

Catana Brown is Associate Professor, University of Kansas Medical Center.

[Haworth co-indexing entry note]: "What Is the Best Environment for Me? A Sensory Processing Perspective." Brown, Catana. Co-published simultaneously in *Occupational Therapy in Mental Health* (The Haworth Press, Inc.) Vol. 17, No. 3/4, 2001, pp. 115-125; and: *Recovery and Wellness: Models of Hope and Empowerment for People with Mental Illness* (ed: Catana Brown) The Haworth Press, Inc., 2001, pp. 115-125. Single or multiple copies of this article are available for a fee from The Haworth Document Delivery Service [1-800-HAWORTH, 9:00 a.m. - 5:00 p.m. (EST). E-mail address: getinfo@haworthpressinc.com].

115

people are having unique experiences and responses to their sensory world. On the other hand if asked questions such as, "Do you like to work in quiet or with background music?" "Do you like to go barefoot?" "Do certain food textures bother you?" or "Do you often ask people to repeat themselves?" most people would have an answer.

Dunn's (1997) Model of Sensory Processing provides a means whereby people can answer these types of questions and in doing so can come to better understand their own sensory processing preferences as well as the preferences of family, friends, and co-workers. Dunn's Model of Sensory Processing along with the corresponding measure, the Adult Sensory Profile, can be part of a recovery toolbox for individuals that are interested in finding ways to better manage their sensory environment. The purpose of this paper is to (1) explain how strategies to manage sensory processing can be related to recovery, (2) describe Dunn's Model of Sensory Processing as a theory for understanding sensory processing, (3) present the Adult Sensory Profile (Brown et al., in press) as a method of assessing sensory processing preferences, (4) discuss sensory processing in psychiatric disability, and (5) identify strategies to support individual sensory processing preferences.

RECOVERY

Recovery is often described as a process that is unique to each individual and involves many phases or components (Deegan, 1996; Young & Ensing, 1999). Stocks (1995) describes the energizing nature of recovery, "I no longer felt pressured to be cured or to be perfect: my only obligation was to be in process" (p. 89). In a study of the process of recovery, Young and Ensing (1999) identified five stages of recovery: overcoming "stuckness, discovering and fostering self-empowerment, learning and self-redefinition, returning to basic functioning and improving quality of life." However, recovery is not a linear process and the experience and stages vary for everyone (Deegan, 1996). The category of returning to basic functioning incorporated many concepts that are generally associated with wellness such as exercise, nutrition, medication monitoring, taking care of living space, doing things I enjoy and connecting with others. Even though there is an explosion of information for the general public related to wellness through venues such as books, workshops, adult education courses and self-help groups, people with mental illness typically have less access to these resources. From a service delivery perspective, psychiatric symptoms tend to be the focus of intervention, often to the exclusion of general health and wellness needs.

Intertwined with recovery is the construct of empowerment (Deegan, 1997). Empowerment involves taking control and responsibility for one's own life. The identification and implementation of individualized coping mechanisms is one of the means by which people can become empowered. Coping mechanisms may target symptoms of mental illness, but should be considered more globally as essential strategies that all people need to manage daily life.

Consequently, to support recovery it is important that people with psychiatric disabilities have access to information and programs that promote wellness and the establishment of effective coping mechanisms. It is also important that the information and programs are available in a consumer-directed manner. This means that the consumer takes an active role in any assessment and intervention procedures and is in control of all decisions regarding the information and/or programs.

In the process of establishing useful coping mechanisms, sensory processing is rarely considered for adults. Understanding personal sensory processing preferences can be a powerful tool to enhance daily life. Self knowledge about sensory processing is empowering as sensory processing preferences can explain an individual's response to particular environments, situations, activities and people. Furthermore, individuals can establish coping strategies and select activities based on an understanding of sensory processing by creating or pursuing environments that best match those preferences.

DUNN'S MODEL OF SENSORY PROCESSING

Dunn's (1997) Model of Sensory Processing describes four types of responses to sensory stimuli based on the intersection of two continua (Table 1). The first continuum is the neurological threshold continuum. The two ends of the continuum are low and high thresholds, though individuals can have responses at any point on the continuum. A low threshold indicates that the nervous system requires less stimuli for the individual to recognize a sensation. Conversely, a high threshold requires more intense sensory stimulation for the neuron to fire and for the individual to recognize the sensation. For example, in the olfactory realm of sensation, the individual with a low threshold registers and distinguishes the different odors of all the foods in the buffet line, while the

TABLE 1. Dunn's Model of Sensory Processing

High Threshold – Behaviors in Accordance **LOW REGISTRATION** Slow to respond, misses cues, easily adaptable to a variety of settings	High Threshold – Behaviors to Counteract **SENSATION SEEKING** Creates sensations, looks for environments rich in sensory stimuli, easily bored
Low Threshold – Behaviors in Accordance **SENSORY SENSITIVITY** Readily notices or aware of sensory features of the environment, distractible	Low Threshold – Behaviors to Counteract **SENSATION AVOIDING** When bothered by stimuli engages in behaviors to limit sensory stimuli, does well with consistency, routine

individual with a high threshold doesn't notice the smells of the food or notices only the most pungent odors.

The second continuum in Dunn's (1997) Model of Sensory Processing is the behavioral response continuum. On this continuum the individual can behave in accordance with the neurological threshold or can engage in behaviors to counteract the neurological threshold. Both behaviors involve a manner of response to the sensation, but the counteractive behaviors require a more deliberate action on the part of the individual to reverse the neurological predisposition.

The intersection of the neurological continuum and the behavioral continuum result in four separate quadrants. These quadrants are construed as independent, so that any combination of quadrant preferences can describe a particular individual's preference in sensory processing. The four quadrants are labeled low registration, sensation seeking, sensory sensitivity and sensation avoiding. All sensory processing preferences typified by the four quadrants have both assets and liabilities. Whether or not a preference is an asset or a liability is dependent upon the task, situation and environment.

Low registration is the quadrant that represents behaviors in accordance with a high neurological threshold. Low registration behaviors are characterized by a slowness to respond or a missing of information. People with low registration may be less aware of things that are happening in their environment that others are noticing. At the same time people with low registration are generally good at tolerating a wide range of environments and can maintain focus on tasks of interest even when distractors are present.

The next quadrant, sensation seeking, is distinguished by behaviors that counteract a high neurological threshold. The sensation seeker creates or pursues environments that are intense enough to cause the neurological system to respond to sensation. Sensation seekers tend to be curious, enjoy novelty and sensory experiences. However, people with high sensation seeking tendencies are easily bored, have difficulty with situations that involve routines and may be uncomfortable or restless in sedate, quiet environments.

Sensory sensitivity is associated with behaviors that are in accordance with a low neurological threshold. Behaviors in this quadrant include a sharp awareness of sensory features in the environment, distractibility, and a tendency to be bothered or overwhelmed by sensory stimulation. People with high sensory sensitivity are inclined towards strong attention to detail and an ability to detect stimuli that others don't notice.

The final quadrant, sensation avoiding, involves behaviors that counteract a low neurological threshold. People with high sensation avoiding find certain sensory stimuli annoying or overwhelming and engage in deliberate behaviors to block exposure to that stimuli. Sensation avoiders typically desire control over situations and therefore prefer consistency and ritual, and have good skills in creating structure or routine.

By way of illustration, imagine the different behaviors that would be typical for each of the four sensory processing preferences during a party with music and dancing. The person with low registration is likely to miss that someone new enters the room, is slow to get a joke but finds it easy to move from situation to situation within the party atmosphere. The sensation seeker is dancing and singing along with the music. The person with sensory sensitivity finds it difficult to focus on a conversation due to all of the distractions, but is good at identifying the ingredients in one of the party dishes. The sensation avoider finds a quiet place in the kitchen to help out and talk one on one with the host.

Contrast the party situation with the same four people attending a lecture. The person with low registration has a tape recorder and is taking lots of notes so that the information can be processed later on. The sensation seeker is chewing gum, wiggling in the chair, and talking to those sitting close by. The sensory sensitive individual admires the detailed overheads of the presenter, but finds it difficult to screen out the sensation seeker seated nearby. The sensation avoider is sitting in the first row on the end and appreciates the structured format and repetition of the speaker.

THE ADULT SENSORY PROFILE

The Adult Sensory Profile (Brown & Dunn, in press) is a measure of sensory processing preferences based on Dunn's (1997) Model of Sensory Processing. It includes four subscales, each with fifteen items representing the quadrants of the model: sensory sensitivity, sensation avoiding, low registration, sensation seeking. The questions reflect behavioral responses to everyday sensory experiences. There are questions for all sensory modalities: visual, auditory, tactile, taste, smell and movement (vestibular and proprioception) with a general category of activity level. It is designed as a self assessment with responses of almost never, rarely, seldom, sometimes, and almost always. Preliminary studies of reliability and validity suggest that the Adult Sensory Profile has promising psychometric properties (Brown et al., 2001; Brown & Dunn, in press), though work in this area is ongoing.

Items in the sensory sensitivity quadrant describe behaviors indicative of discomfort with stimuli or distractibility, while items in the sensation avoiding quadrant reflect active efforts to diminish stimuli. Items in poor registration are illustrated by a lack of detection of stimuli, and sensation seeking items involve active engagement with the sensory environment.

The Adult Sensory Profile was developed so that it can be self-administered and self-scored or can be used with the support of a service provider. After completing the measure, a score is tabulated for each of the four quadrants, sensory sensitivity, sensation avoiding, low registration and sensation seeking. After computing a score, the individual can compare his/her score with average scores for the quadrants. This comparison allows for a determination as to whether a particular score is higher or lower than average, so for example the individual can assess if the score suggests, "I tend to avoid sensation more than most people, the same as most people or less than most people." The scoring also allows the individual to look within particular sensory modalities. A score may be average, but there may be particular areas that stand out. For example, someone with an average sensory sensitivity score may find a particular sensitivity in the touch realm.

Any pattern of scores is possible, and it is understanding the pattern of scores that can be most informative. For example, someone with high sensory sensitivity scores and low sensation avoiding scores suggests that although the person easily notices, responds and has a tendency to be distracted and overwhelmed by sensation (high sensory sensitivity), this person rarely engages in behaviors to restrict the environment (low sensation avoiding). This individual may find that he/she can more easily participate in daily activities by employing strategies that reduce sensory stimulation. Even patterns that seem contradictory can exist. For example, some individuals have high scores in both the sensation seeking and sensation avoiding quadrants indicating that this person is inclined to take control of the sensory environment and is intentional about either increasing or diminishing available sensory stimuli.

SENSORY PROCESSING
AND PEOPLE WITH PSYCHIATRIC DISABILITIES

Before discussing sensory processing and psychiatric disabilities, it is important to note that Dunn's (1997) Model of Sensory Processing is not intended to identify pathology. All individuals have patterns of sensory processing preferences and there is a great deal of heterogeneity among all adults. However, it is possible that certain preferences may be associated with certain experiences associated with psychiatric disability. The Adult Sensory Profile was used in a research study to examine differences in sensory processing for people with schizophrenia, people with bipolar disorder and people without mental illness (Brown, 1999). This study indicated that people with schizophrenia tended to have sensory processing preferences for both sensation avoiding and low registration. People with bipolar disorder had preferences for sensation avoiding and people without mental illness were characterized primarily by sensation seeking behavior. However, it is important to note that there is a large variability among groups, so that any one individual does not necessarily fit the pattern. In fact, the greatest variability existed in the group of people with schizophrenia. In addition, this single study needs replication to enhance confidence in these findings.

Understanding sensory processing for people with psychiatric disabilities is also enhanced through personal narratives. The salience of sensory processing and psychiatric disability becomes clear with the frequency of first person accounts that include descriptions of personal sensory experiences. In a now classic description of interviews with people with schizophrenia, McGhie and Chapman (1961) analyzed statements related to the personal experience of perception. Some of the quotes suggest distractibility. "My concentration is very poor. I jump from one thing to another. If I am talking to someone, they only need to cross their legs or scratch their heads and I am distracted and forget what I was saying. I think I could concentrate better with my eyes shut"

(p. 104). Others suggest an increased intensity. "During the last while back I have noticed that noises all seem to be louder to me than they were before. It's as if someone had turned up the volume" (p. 105). Both of these types of experiences would be consistent with the construct of sensory sensitivity. Other quotes describe experiences conforming to the low registration construct. "I'm slow in everything and everything is too quick for me to pick up. It's not that they talk too fast, it's me that's slow" (p. 106). "Everything is in bits. You put the picture up bit by bit into your head . . . If I move there's a new picture that I have to put together again" (p. 106).

As the appreciation for first person accounts of individuals with psychiatric disabilities has grown, there are many more opportunities to learn from these stories. Both Weingarten (1989) and Leete (1989) have shared experiences of living with a psychiatric disability and corresponding strategies for managing difficult situations. They express remarkably similar reactions related to encountering new situations. Leete (1989) says, "There are enormous pressures that come with any new experience or new environment, and any change, positive or negative is extremely difficult" (p. 199). Weingarten (1989) expresses similar sentiments and describes how he attempts to manage the difficulty. "I feel enormous pressure when I encounter new experiences, environments and people, so it is easy for me to become overstimulated at these times. I've learned to overcome these situations by (1) avoiding them when possible, and (2) going back to them until I mastered them" (p. 639). Frese (1993) offers his strategy. "I find that when I begin to become overstimulated, it is often helpful to politely excuse myself and withdraw from the situation" (p. 43).

Other comments from first person accounts reflect slowness or difficulty in making sense or meaning of information or the environment. "When I am blocked by confusion, or a total scrambling of my thoughts, interjections of obtuse phrases, and coded associations I cannot explain, I can only go through it and accept it as what my brain does" (Ruocchio, 1991). Payne (1992) offers a particularly striking depiction. "I felt as though I had been pushed deep within myself, and I had little or no reaction to events or emotions around me . . . Everything outside of me seemed to fade into the distance; everything was miles away from me" (Payne, 1992).

STRATEGIES

From the first person accounts just described, it is clear that people tend to develop their own coping mechanisms to manage their sensory processing experiences. Narratives provide insights into strategies that can be useful for many. However, it is possible to enhance or develop more effective strategies if one has an expanded understanding of sensory processing. Based on Dunn's (1997) Model of Sensory Processing, the approach to intervention focuses on identifying or adapting environments that support the sensory processing preferences of the individual. An assumption of the model is that each individual has a comfort range in which he/she functions. Individuals can sometimes find strategies to extend that range, but in most situations the most satisfying and effective approach will target the environment. In some cases, the same strategy may be utilized for two different preferences, but the reason for employing the strategy is different. For example, it can be useful for people with both sensory sensitivity and low registration to talk through a task. With sensory sensitivity this strategy can help the person stay focused, while in low registration, the strategy provides a cue to support processing of information.

Once an individual is aware of sensory processing preferences, that individual is better able to utilize strategies to create environments and situations that support those preferences. In fact, awareness, in and of itself, is empowering. It helps the individual to understand why he/she responds in certain ways to certain situations, and why others may respond differently. For example, it may help the sensation avoider to understand why he/she likes to read in a quiet place, while a sensation seeking friend keeps the television on while reading. It also can be very helpful in identifying potentially difficult situations and in using this information to prepare for the situation. Orrin (1994) describes how awareness is helpful to her. "The recognition of individual needs, for me, has also included the awareness of the importance for me to listen to my body . . . I am referring to my own internal flow. I have discovered that I know when I want to be with a friend, when I want to browse through a store, when I want to write or go for a walk, when I want to work on a project or a therapy exercise . . . By listening to myself, and following the promptings that come from myself, I find that I am happier" (p. 44).

In occupational therapy intervention, it is important to first identify what the person wants or needs to do. Then specific intervention strategies can be identified to support performance. These strategies focus on adapting the environment or making the best person-environment match rather than changing a person's sensory processing.

Generally, each sensory processing preference suggests particularly types of strategies. Specific suggestions for strategies are outlined in the

Adolescent/Adult Sensory Profile Manual (Brown & Dunn, in press). For the low threshold preferences of sensory sensitivity and sensation avoiding, strategies are used that organize or reduce sensory stimuli. In sensory sensitivity, the emphasis is on strategies that help the individual stay focused, screen out irrelevant information and pick up on important information. With this preference the individual may be reactive and/or distractible, but does not necessarily want to withdraw from the sensory environment. Therefore, strategies that organize or systematize information may be helpful. With sensation avoiding, the preference is to withdraw. In this case, strategies involve eliminating excess stimuli and incorporating acceptable methods of escaping overwhelming situations.

With the high threshold preferences of low registration and sensation seeking there is an emphasis on enhancing or increasing the sensory stimuli. In low registration, the individual can benefit from strategies that make information obvious or ensure that sensory processing has occurred. In sensation seeking, sensory stimuli is added or intensified to meet sensory needs.

CONCLUSION

An appreciation for sensory processing preferences can provide consumers with psychiatric disabilities practical information to support empowerment and wellness. The strategies addressing sensory processing preferences can be utilized by consumers and occupational therapists in several ways. Consumers can identify strategies that work best for their individual needs. Consumers can inform occupational therapists, other service providers and other consumers about effective strategies that they have developed. There is a great deal of untapped knowledge that can be garnered from the lived experiences of people with psychiatric disabilities.

Occupational therapists may use the strategies described in this paper as well as others learned from consumers or their own practice to enhance existing intervention approaches. For example, in a grocery shopping intervention program developed by the author and colleagues, strategies are used that increase the salience of the existing cues in the grocery store to compensate for potential low registration (e.g., participants practice using overhead signs to help locate an item). Occupational therapists may also use the strategies when providing recommendations for best fitting activities and environments and/or actually assisting with or providing environmental adaptations. For example, in a work setting, the steps for a particular job were written out to support an individual having difficulty processing auditory information. From a population perspective, occupational therapists can help design or adapt service and community settings to support particular sensory processing needs. To illustrate, an occupational therapist used knowledge of sensory processing to design a relaxation room at a community support program for individuals with high sensory sensitivity.

Life involves a constant encounter with the sensory world. Increasing awareness of particular responses to that encounter is empowering. It gives the means by which people can seek out or adapt environments that are more supportive of their own particular needs. In so doing people move from being dominated by their environments and to a position of mastery.

REFERENCES

Brown, C., Tollefson, N., Dunn, W., Cromwell, R., & Filion, D., (in press). The Adult Sensory Profile: Measuring patterns of sensory processing. *American Journal of Occupational Therapy, 55*, 75-82.

Brown, C. & Dunn, W. (in press). *The Adolescent/Adult Sensory Profile Manual.* Psychological Corporation.

Deegan, P. (1996). Recovery as a journey of the heart. *Psychiatric Rehabilitation Journal, 19*(3), 91-97.

Deegan, P.E. (1997). Recovery and empowerment for people with psychiatric disabilities. *Social Work in Mental Health: Trends and Issues, 25*, 11-24.

Frese, F.J. (1993). Twelve aspect of coping for persons with serious and persistent mental illness. *Innovations and Research 2*(3), 39-46.

Leete, E. (1989). How I perceive and mange my illness. *Schizophrenia Bulletin, 15*, 197-200.

McGhie, A. & Chapman, J. (1961). Disorders of attention and perception in early schizophrenia. *British Journal of Medical Psychology, 34*, 103-116.

Orrin, D. (1994). Past the struggles of mental illness, toward the development of quality lives. *Innovations and Research, 3*(3), 41-45.

Payne, R.L. (1992). My schizophrenia. *Schizophrenia Bulletin, 18*, 725-728.

Ruocchio, P.J. (1991). The schizophrenic inside. *Schizophrenia Bulletin, 17*, 357-360.

Stock, M.L. (1995). In the eye of the beholder. *Psychiatric Rehabilitation Journal, 19*(1), 89–91.

Weingarten, R. (1989). How I've managed chronic mental illness. *Schizophrenia Bulletin, 15*, 635-640.

Young, S.L. & Ensing, D.S. (1999). Exploring recovery from the perspective of people with psychiatric disabilities. *Psychiatric Rehabilitation Journal, 22*(3), 219-231.

Wellness Recovery Action Plan: A System for Monitoring, Reducing and Eliminating Uncomfortable or Dangerous Physical Symptoms and Emotional Feelings

Mary Ellen Copeland, MS, MA

SUMMARY. This article describes a popular and effective self monitoring and response system that was developed in 1997 by 30 people who attended an eight day mental health recovery skills seminar in Vermont. They developed the system in response to their need for a structured way to use their wellness tools to relieve and eliminate their symptoms, and to stay well. While it was developed by and for people who are dealing with troubling emotional symptoms, the Wellness Recovery Action Plan can be used by anyone to deal with any kind of physical or emotional illness or issue. People who use the plan develop it by identifying tools or responses that will help them to relieve symptoms and/or enhance their wellness. They then use these tools to develop a Wellness Recovery Action Plan that includes: (1) a daily maintenance list, (2) identifying and responding to triggers, (3) identifying and responding to early warning signs, (4) recognizing when things are getting much worse and responding in ways that will help them feel better and (5) a crisis plan or ad-

Mary Ellen Copeland is a teacher, writer and lecturer from Brattleboro, VT. She is the author of the *Depression Workbook, Winning Against Relapse,* and the Wellness Recovery Action Plan.

[Haworth co-indexing entry note]: "Wellness Recovery Action Plan: A System for Monitoring, Reducing and Eliminating Uncomfortable or Dangerous Physical Symptoms and Emotional Feelings." Copeland, Mary Ellen. Co-published simultaneously in *Occupational Therapy in Mental Health* (The Haworth Press, Inc.) Vol. 17, No. 3/4, 2001, pp. 127-150; and: *Recovery and Wellness: Models of Hope and Empowerment for People with Mental Illness* (ed: Catana Brown) The Haworth Press, Inc., 2001, pp. 127-150. Single or multiple copies of this article are available for a fee from The Haworth Document Delivery Service [1-800-HAWORTH, 9:00 a.m. - 5:00 p.m. (EST). E-mail address: getinfo@haworthpressinc.com].

127

vanced directive. The people who developed this plan emphasize that the plan must be developed by the person who will use it, although they can reach out to their supporters for assistance. *[Article copies available for a fee from The Haworth Document Delivery Service: 1-800-HAWORTH. E-mail address: <getinfo@haworthpressinc.com> Website: <http://www.HaworthPress. com> © 2001 by The Haworth Press, Inc. All rights reserved.]*

KEYWORDS. Self management, self help, mental health, psychiatric symptoms, mental illness

The Wellness Recovery Action Plan is an amazingly effective individualized, self help system that is being widely used by people who experience psychiatric symptoms to promote their recovery. It was developed by a group of about thirty people that included people who experience psychiatric symptoms, family members and care providers. I had been working with this group for about eight days, teaching them self help skills and tools, when one of the group members said, "This is all great, but I have no idea how to structure it into my life. I am very disorganized and have never been able to do anything consistently." Others agreed. So we began working together to develop a system that would facilitate incorporating the use of these skills and strategies into everyday life. With lots of hard work and "trial and error" the group members came up with a system that people are finding works for them.

The positive response to this system has been overwhelming. It is now being used to enhance and support the wellness process by individuals and groups, health care agencies and hospitals around the world. While it was specifically developed to be used by people who experience psychiatric symptoms, people with all kinds of health conditions, and even some who have no significant complaints but want to stay healthy, have found this system to be of value. I use it consistently myself. It works very well for me. When things are starting to "go down the drain," my husband says, "Where's the blue book?"

I have described this plan at workshops and conferences and the response is always the same. "This is something I can do for myself, something that will work." This article will give an overview of WRAP, specific directions for developing a WRAP and ideas for working with individuals and groups in developing WRAP plans.

OVERVIEW

The Wellness Recovery Action Program is a structured system for monitoring uncomfortable and distressing symptoms and, through planned responses, reducing, modifying or eliminating those symptoms. It also includes plans for responses from others when a person's symptoms have made it impossible to continue to make decisions, take care of him/herself and keep him/herself safe. Anecdotal reporting from people who are using this system indicates that it is working for them by helping them to feel better more often and by improving the overall quality of their life. The activities involved in developing this plan help people to focus on their strengths and gives them a strong sense of personal responsibility and empowerment.

Using a three ring binder, a set of tabs or dividers, and lined three ring paper, a five part system is developed by the person who experiences the symptoms. People completing the plan may be assisted in the process by the supporters and health care professionals *of their choice* but, to be effective and empowering, *the person experiencing the symptoms must develop the plan for himself/herself.*

The planning process begins by developing a Wellness Toolbox, a listing of skills and strategies that the person has used or wants to use to keep well and to feel better when not well.

Section 1 is a Daily Maintenance List. Part 1 is a description of how the person feels when feeling well. Part 2 is a list of everything the person needs to do every day to maintain wellness. Part 3 is a list of things the person might need to consider doing that day.

Section 2 deals with triggers. Part 1 identifies those events or situations which, if they occur, might cause uncomfortable symptoms to begin. Part 2 is a plan of "What to Do" if any of these triggers occur.

Section 3 deals with early warning signs. Part 1 involves identification of those subtle signs that may indicate that the situation is beginning to worsen. Part 2 is a plan of "What to Do" if any of these early warning signs are noticed.

Section 4 deals with symptoms that occur when the situation has gotten much worse but has not yet reached a crisis, where the person can still take action in their own behalf. Part 2 is a plan of "What to Do" if any of these symptoms occur.

Section 5 is multifaceted. It identifies those symptoms that indicate a person can no longer continue to make decisions, take care of himself/herself and keep himself/herself safe. It is for use by supporters and health care professionals on behalf of the person that developed the plan. Part 1 is information that defines what the person is like when well. Part 2 identifies those symptoms that indicate others need to take over responsibility for the person's care. Part 3 names those supporters and identifies their roles. Part 4 identifies those medications which, if necessary, are all right with the person, those which are not, and the reasons why. Part 5 gives the person the option of developing a home, community care or respite center plan to use, if possible, instead of hospitalization. Part 6 identifies the treatment facilities which, if necessary, are all right with the person, those which are not, and the reasons why. Part 7 identifies the treatments which, if necessary, are all right with the person, those which are not, and the reasons why. Part 8 is an intensive description of what is wanted from supporters–and what is not wanted–when symptoms become this intense. Part 9 gives information for supporters to use in determining when the person no longer needs their supporters to use this crisis plan.

GETTING STARTED

All that is needed to develop a WRAP is:

1. a three ring binder, one inch thick will do–a two or four ring binder will work as well
2. a set of five dividers or tabs
3. a package of three ring filler paper, most people preferred lined
4. a writing instrument of some kind
5. (optional) a friend, health care provider or other supporter to give assistance and feedback

Some people prefer to use a computer to develop their system. The pages can be printed on three ring binder paper or punched with three holes. If a person does not like to write or cannot write, the person could ask someone else to do the writing. Responses could also be tape recorded.

STEP 1. DEVELOPING A WELLNESS TOOLBOX

The first step in developing a Wellness Recovery Action Plan, is to develop a Wellness Toolbox. This is a listing of things a person has done in the past, or could do, to stay well; and, things that could be done to help the person feel better when they are not doing well. The person will use these "tools" to develop his/her own WRAP. This list is kept in the front of the binder for easy reference as a person is developing the plan.

On one of several sheets of paper inserted in the front of the binder, the person lists the tools, strategies and skills used regularly to keep well, along with those used frequently or occasionally to feel better and to relieve troubling symptoms. This includes tools used in the past, things the person heard of and thought he/she might like to try, and things that have been recommended by health care providers and other supporters. The person can get ideas on other tools from self-help books including those by Mary Ellen Copeland: *The Depression Workbook: A Guide to Living With Depression and Manic Depression; Living Without Depression and Manic Depression: A Guide to Maintaining Mood Stability; Depression; The Worry Control Workbook; Winning Against Relapse; Healing the Trauma of Abuse;* and *The Loneliness Workbook.* The audio tapes *Winning Against Relapse Program* and *Strategies for Living with Depression and Manic Depression* may also be helpful. Strategizing about these tools is an excellent group activity. People get ideas on things to do to help themselves from each other. Working together in this way, people often come up with very long lists of tools.

The following is list that includes some tools that are most commonly used to stay well and help relieve symptoms:

1. Talk to a friend or health care professional
2. Peer counseling or exchange listening
3. Focusing exercises
4. Relaxation and stress reduction exercises
5. Guided imagery
6. Journaling–writing in a notebook
7. Creative, affirming and/or diversionary activities
8. Exercise
9. Diet considerations
10. Light through your eyes
11. Extra rest
12. Time off from home or work responsibilities
13. Take medications, vitamins, minerals, herbal supplements
14. Attend a support group
15. Do something "normal" like washing your hair, shaving or going to work

16. Get a medication check
17. Get a second opinion
18. Call a warm or hot line
19. Wear something that makes you feel good
20. Look through old pictures, scrapbooks and photo albums
21. Make a list of your accomplishments
22. Spend ten minutes writing down everything good you can think of about yourself
23. Do something that makes you laugh or something special for someone else
24. Repeat positive affirmations
25. Focus on and appreciate what is happening right now
26. Listen to music, make music or sing

This list of tools could also include things the person would want to avoid like:

1. alcohol, sugar and caffeine
2. going to bars
3. getting over-tired
4. certain people

STEP 2. DAILY MAINTENANCE LIST

The Daily Maintenance List is a list of things that the person feels need to be done *every day* to maintain their wellness. Writing them down and then reminding oneself to do these things each day is often the most important step toward wellness. A daily maintenance plan helps the person recognize those things which need to be done to remain healthy, and then to plan each day so that these things are included. While this Daily Maintenance List may seem silly or simplistic to some people, many people feel that, by attending to this list, they have made great strides in their recovery. The person developing the plan writes Daily Maintenance List on the first tab and inserts it in the binder followed by several sheets of filler paper.

The first page is a reminder list of how the person feels when well. For a person that has not been feeling well, this list is an important reference point. The person describes what he/she is like when feeling fine or OK–usually in list form. Some descriptive words that others have used include bright, cheerful, talkative, outgoing, boisterous, happy, flamboyant, athletic, optimistic, reasonable, responsible, competent, capable, industrious and curious. If the person says he/she never felt well or can't remember ever feeling well, the person might list those words that describe how he/she would like to feel.

On the next page, using the wellness toolbox as a reference, the person makes a list of things they know they need to do every day to maintain their wellness. For many people this is the most important part of their plan. It is important that the plan is "do-able" or it can become another frustration. This list can be short or long–depending on the person's needs and abilities. Some ideas for this plan include:

- eat three healthy meals and three healthy snacks
- drink at least six-8 ounce glasses of water
- avoid caffeine, sugar, junk foods, alcohol
- exercise for at least 1/2 hour
- get exposure to outdoor light for at least 1/2 hour
- take medications and vitamin supplements
- have 20 minutes of relaxation or meditation time
- write in my journal for at least 15 minutes
- spend at least 1/2 hour enjoying a fun, affirming and/or creative activity
- get support from a friend
- check in with my partner for at least 10 minutes
- check in with myself: how am I doing physically, emotionally, mentally and spiritually

On the next page, the person can make a reminder list for things that need to be done. Reading through this list daily helps keep the person on track, relieving stress. Some ideas for this list include things like:

- spend time with my counselor or case manager
- set up an appointment with one of my health care professionals
- spend time with a good friend or with my partner
- be in touch with my family
- spend time with children or pets
- do peer counseling
- get more sleep
- do some housework
- buy groceries
- do the laundry
- have some personal time

- plan something fun for the weekend or the evening
- write some letters
- remember someone's birthday or anniversary
- go out for a long walk or do some other extended outdoor activity (gardening, fishing, etc.)

That's the first section of the book. It can be changed or rewritten whenever the person who wrote it feels that is necessary. This section should be reviewed daily until the person using it easily remembers the items on the list.

STEP 3. TRIGGERS

Triggers are external events or circumstances that, if they happen, may produce symptoms that are, or may be, very uncomfortable. These symptoms often make a person feel like he/she is getting ill. These are normal reactions to life events, but if they are not addressed, these triggers may actually cause symptoms or a worsening in symptoms. The awareness of this susceptibility and development of plans to deal with triggering events when they come up increases the ability to cope, and prevents the development of an acute episode. *It is not important to project catastrophic things that might happen, such as war, natural disaster, or a huge personal loss. If those things were to occur, the person would use the actions described in the triggers action plan more often and/or increase the length of time they are used. The triggers listed here should be those that are more likely to occur.*

On the next tab the person writes "Triggers" and puts in several sheets of binder paper. On the first page, the person writes those things that, if they happened, might cause an increase in symptoms. They may have triggered or increased symptoms in the past.

Triggers include things like:

- the anniversary dates of losses or trauma
- traumatic news events
- being very over-tired
- work stress
- family friction
- a relationship ending
- spending too much time alone
- being judged, criticized, teased or put-down

- financial problems
- physical illness
- sexual harassment or inappropriate sexual behavior
- hateful outbursts by others
- aggressive-sounding noises (sustained)
- being a scapegoat
- reminders of abandonment or deprivation
- self blame
- extreme guilt (from saying "No," etc.)
- substance abuse

On the next page, using the Wellness Toolbox, the person develops a plan of what can be done if triggers interfere with wellness. One person came up with the following plan: "If any of my triggers come up, I will do the following":

- make sure I do everything on my daily maintenance program
- call a support person and ask them to listen while I talk through the situation
- do some deep breathing exercises
- take good care of myself in every way
- work on changing negative thoughts to positive
- get validation from someone I feel close to
- meditate for half an hour

In addition, if I had time, I could:

- write in my journal
- go for a walk
- do some focusing exercises
- have peer counseling session
- see or talk to my counselor, case manager or sponsor
- take a time-out in a comfortable place
- play my musical instrument

STEP 4. EARLY WARNING SIGNS

Early warning signs are internal and may be unrelated to reactions to stressful situations. In spite of the person's best efforts at reducing symptoms, he/she may begin to experience early warning signs, subtle signs of change that indicate a need to take some further action. Recognizing early warning signs and reviewing them regularly will help the person to become more aware of these early warning signs, allowing the person to take action before the signs worsen.

On the next tab the person writes "Early Warning Signs," following that tab with several sheets of lined paper. On the first page the person writes a list of early warning signs noticed in previous situations. The person may want to ask friends, family members and health care providers for early warning signs that they've noticed. Some early warning signs that others have reported include:

- anxiety
- nervousness
- forgetfulness
- the inability to experience pleasure
- lack of motivation
- feeling slowed down or speeded up
- being uncaring
- avoiding others or isolating
- being obsessed with something that doesn't really matter
- the beginning of irrational thought patterns–feeling unconnected to my body
- increased irritability and negativity
- an increase in smoking
- impulsivity
- feelings of discouragement and hopelessness
- feeling worthless, inadequate
- being too quiet
- being easily frustrated

The next page or pages are for developing a plan for responding to these early warning signs in ways to relieve them and to prevent them from worsening. Using the ideas in the appendix and other techniques discovered on their own, the person develops a plan they can follow when these symptoms occur. The following is a sample plan:

Things I Must Do:

- do the things on my daily maintenance plan whether I feel like it or not
- tell a supporter/counselor how I am feeling, ask for the person's advice and to help me figure out how to take the action suggested.

- peer counsel at least once a day until early warning signs diminish
- do at least one focusing exercise a day until early warning signs diminish
- do at least three 10 minute relaxation exercises each day until early warning signs diminish
- write in my journal for at least 15 minutes each day until early warning signs diminish
- spend at least 1 hour involved in an activity I enjoy each day until early warning signs diminish
- ask others to take over my household responsibilities for a day

Other things I could choose to do if they feel right to me:

- check in with my physician or other health care professional
- spend some time with my pet(s)
- read a good book
- dance, sing, listen to good music, play a musical instrument
- exercise
- go fishing

STEP 5. THINGS ARE BREAKING DOWN OR GETTING WORSE

In spite of the best efforts of the person who is experiencing the symptoms, these symptoms may progress to the point where they are very uncomfortable, serious and even dangerous, *but the person is still able to take some action on his/her own behalf.* This is a very important time. It is necessary to take immediate action to prevent a crisis.

On the next tab the person writes, "When Things Are Breaking Down" or some other words that mean the person is having a very difficult time. Then the person makes a list of the symptoms which, for that person, mean things have worsened and are close to the crisis stage. These symptoms vary from person to person. What may mean "things are breaking down to one person" may mean a "crisis" to another. Some symptoms that might be included in this list include:

- feeling very oversensitive and fragile
- irrational responses to events and the actions of others
- feeling very needy
- unable to sleep for (specify for how long)

- increased pain
- headaches
- sleeping all the time
- avoiding eating
- wanting to be totally alone
- racing thoughts
- risk-taking behaviors, e.g., driving fast
- thoughts of self-harm
- substance abuse
- being obsessed with negative thoughts
- inability to slow down
- excessive spending
- bizarre behaviors
- dissociation (blacking out, spacing out, losing time)
- seeing things that aren't there
- taking out anger on others
- chain smoking
- spending excessive amounts of money (say how much that means for you)
- substance abuse
- food abuse
- NOT feeling
- suicidal thoughts
- paranoia

On the next page, the person writes a plan that he/she thinks will help reduce symptoms when progressed to this point. The plan now needs to be very directive with fewer choices and very clear instructions. The following is a sample plan:

If these symptoms come up I need to do *all* of the following:

- call my doctor or other health care professional; ask for and follow his/her instructions
- call and talk as long as I need to my supporters
- arrange for someone to stay with me around the clock until my symptoms subside
- take action so I cannot hurt myself if my symptoms get worse, such as give my medications, check book, credit cards and car keys to a previously designated friend for safe keeping
- make sure I am doing everything on my daily check list

- arrange and take at least three days off from any responsibilities
- have at least two peer counseling sessions daily
- do three deep breathing relaxation exercises daily
- do two focusing exercises each day
- write in my journal for at least one half hour each day

Other choices for the day might include:

- creative activities
- exercise

Ask myself, do I need:

- a physical examination
- to have medications checked

STEP 6. CRISIS PLANNING

Noticing and responding to symptoms early reduces the chances that a person will find himself/herself in crisis. But it is important to confront the possibility of crisis, because *in spite of best planning and assertive action, a person could be in a situation where others will need to take over responsibility for the person's care. This is a difficult situation, one that no one likes to face. In a crisis the person may feel totally out of control. If the person writes a clear crisis plan when feeling well, to instruct others about how to be cared for when not well, this keeps the person in control even when it seems like things are out of control.* It will keep family members and friends from wasting time trying to figure out what to do that will be helpful. It relieves the guilt felt by family members and other caregivers who may have wondered whether they were taking the right action. It also insures that critical needs will be met and that the person will get better as quickly as possible.

A crisis plan needs to be developed by the person when feeling well. However, it cannot be done quickly. The person can work at it for a while, then leave it for several days and keep coming back to it until the person feels the plan has the best chance of working. Decisions like this take time, thought and often collaboration with health care providers, family members and other supporters. Information that others have used in crisis plans may be useful to a person who is developing such a plan for the first time.

The crisis plan differs from the other action plans in that it will be used by others. The other four sections of this planning process are usually implemented by the person who developed the plan and need not be shared with anyone else unless the person wants to do that. It can be written language that only the person who wrote it needs to understand. A crisis plan needs to be written so that it is clear, legible and easy for others to understand the intention of the person developing the document. When the plan is completed, copies should be given to the people named as supporters.

On the next tab the person writes Crisis Plan and inserts it in the binder followed by several pieces of lined paper.

Part 1: What I'm Like When I'm Feeling Well

The first step in this process is describing what the person feels like when well. While family and friends know what the person is like, an emergency room doctor may mistake personality traits for symptoms. This could result in poor decision making or mistreatment. This first part of the Crisis Plan could easily be copied from the first section of the Daily Maintenance List.

Part 2: Symptoms

Many people find that this is the most difficult part of developing the crisis plan. It is very hard to think back over previous episodes to try and figure out those symptoms that would indicate to others that they need to take over responsibility for the person's care and make decisions on the person's behalf. This is hard for everyone. No one likes to think that anyone will ever have to take over responsibility for his/her self and care. And yet, through careful, well developed descriptions, a person can stay in control even when things seem to be out of control.

A person should take as much time as they need to complete this section. When the person starts to feel discouraged or daunted, he/she should set it aside for awhile. Input can be requested from friends, family members and health care professionals. *However, the final determination must be the person who experiences the symptoms.* Symptoms might include:

- unable to recognize or incorrectly identifying family members and friends
- unconscious or semi-conscious

- uncontrollable pacing, unable to stay still, very rapid breathing or seeming to be gasping for breath
- severe agitated depression
- unable to stop repeating very negative statements like "I want to die"
- inability to stop compulsive behaviors like constantly counting everything
- catatonic–unmoving for long periods of time
- neglecting personal hygiene (for days)
- not cooking or doing any housework (for days)
- extreme mood swings daily
- destructive to property (throwing things, etc.)
- not understanding what people are saying
- thinking I am someone I am not
- thinking I have the ability to do something I don't
- self destructive behavior
- abusive or violent behavior
- criminal activities
- substance abuse
- threatening suicide or acting suicidal
- not getting out of bed at all
- refusing to eat or drink

Part 3: Supporters

The next section of the crisis plan lists those people who the person wants to take over for them when the symptoms they list occur. It is suggested that a person have at least five people on their list of supporters. If they have only one or two, the supporters might not be available when they are needed. They can be family members, friends or health care professionals. (If they do not now have five supporters, they should list those they do have and add to the list as they develop new supports.) Again, in order to increase the likelihood that this plan will work, this must be a list of people that the person who is developing the plan chooses. Initially, this may be mostly health care professionals. But as the person works on other areas of their recovery including a strong support system, they may come to rely more heavily on the natural supports of family members and friends. Using natural supports is less expensive, less invasive and normal. Following are some examples of attributes people want from those who take over and make decisions for them:

- responsible
- honest
- sincere
- knowledgeable
- calm
- compassionate
- understanding
- trustworthy

The following format may be used in listing supporters:

Name   Connection/role   Phone number

Specific tasks

There may be health care professionals or family members that have
made decisions that were not according to the person's wishes in the
past. They could inadvertently get involved in the person's care again.
This can be prevented by including the following section in the plan.

I *do not* want the following people involved in any way in my care or
treatment:

Name   Why you do not want them involved (optional)

Many people like to include a section that describes how possible
disputes between supporters be settled. For instance, the person may
want to say that a majority need to agree, or that a particular person or
two people make the determination in that case. Or the person may want
some organization or agency to intervene on their behalf.

Part 4: Medication

The medication section includes the name of the person's physician
and/or other health care providers (including their area of expertise and
phone number), their pharmacy (including phone number) and lists of:

- allergies
- medications the person is currently using and why taking them
- those medications the person would prefer to take if medications
  or additional medications became necessary and why the person
  would choose those

- those medications that should be avoided and why they should be avoided

Part 5: Treatments

In this section the person lists preferred treatments and treatments to be avoided. Many people have very strong feelings about electroshock therapy and other therapy options–both positive and negative. The person needs to be sure supporters know his/her feelings and preferences regarding treatment. The reason may be as simple as "This treatment has or has not worked in the past," or the person may have some other reasons for refusing such a treatment. This list can include therapies like acupuncture, massage therapy, homeopathy.

Part 6: Home/Community Care/Respite Center

Many people are setting up plans so that they can stay at home and still get the care they need if they are in a crisis by having around the clock care from supporters and regular visits with health care professionals. Community care and respite centers are being set up around the country as an alternative to hospitalization where a person can be supported by peers until symptoms subside. The person may need to talk with others about this and explore options that are available in his/her community. Then the person should describe in the plan exactly what he/she wants to happen. The person may need to make some arrangements to make sure the designated wishes can be followed.

Part 7: Treatment Facilities

When supporters cannot provide needed care at home or in the community, a safe hospital treatment facility may be needed. The person develops a list of acceptable facilities, using personal experience and information learned through research or through talking with others. The person should also list those places to be avoided.

Part 8: Help from Others

The next section describes what others can do to be helpful when a person is in a crisis. This takes a lot of thought. Supporters and other health care professionals can help by sharing ideas. Some ideas include:

- listen to me without giving me advice, judging me or criticizing me
- hold me
- let me pace
- encourage me to move, help me move
- lead me through a relaxation or stress reduction technique
- peer counsel with me
- take me for a walk
- provide me with materials so I can draw or paint
- give me the space to express my feelings
- don't talk to me (or do talk to me)
- encourage me
- reassure me
- feed me good food
- make sure I get exposure to outdoor light for at least 1/2 hour daily
- play me comic videos
- play me good music (list the kind)
- just let me rest
- keep me from hurting myself, even if that means you have to restrain me or get help from others
- keep me from being abusive to, or hurting others, do whatever you have to do to keep me from doing that

Specific tasks that others need to do along with the name of the specific person or people to do this task should also be listed. This includes things like:

- child, pet and plant care
- buying groceries
- paying bills including the rent or mortgage
- taking care of housekeeping tasks
- doing the laundry
- cooking

Include a listing of things that others should not do because they would not help, might worsen symptoms or be harmful. Some examples include:

- trying to entertain me or divert my attention
- chattering
- certain kinds of music

- certain videos
- getting angry with me
- impatience
- invalidation
- not being heard

Part 9: When Supporters No Longer Need to Use This Plan

It is expected that the person will feel better very soon. Supporters will no longer need to follow this plan to keep the person safe. Include here a listing, developed by the person who will use the plan, of indicators that supporters no longer need to follow this plan. Some examples include:

- when I have slept through the night for three nights
- when I eat at least two good meals a day
- when I am always reasonable and rational
- when I am taking care of my personal hygiene needs
- when I can carry on a good conversation
- when I keep my living space organized
- when I can be in a crowd without being anxious

This plan should be updated whenever the person learns new information or changes his/her mind about things. Supporters are given new copies each time it is revised.

It will help assure that this crisis plan will be followed if it is notarized and signed in the presence of two witnesses. It will further increase its potential for use if the person appoints a durable power of attorney. Since the legality of these documents varies from state to state, it is not possible to know if the plan will be followed. However, it is the person's best assurance that his/her wishes will be honored.

HOW TO USE WRAP

In order to use this program successfully, at first the person will have to be willing to spend up to 15 or 20 minutes daily reviewing the pages, and be willing to take action if indicated. Most people report that morning, either before or after breakfast, is the best time to review the book. As the person becomes familiar with the symptoms and plans, he/she will find that the review process takes less time and that the person will know how to respond to certain symptoms without even referring to the book.

The person can begin by reviewing the first page in Section 1, Daily Maintenance Plan, "How you are if you are all right." If the person is all right, the person refers to the list of things you need to do every day to keep yourself well during that day. The person should also refer to the page of things the person may need to do to see if anything else needs to be done. If it does, the person makes a note to include it in the day.

If the person is not feeling alright, he/she reviews the other sections to see where the symptoms being experienced fit in. Then the person follows the action plan that he/she designed.

For instance, if the person feels very anxious because the person got a big bill in the mail or had an argument with a spouse, the person follows the plan in the triggers section. If the person notices some early warning signs (subtle signs that symptoms might be worsening), like forgetting things or avoiding answering the phone, the person follows the plan designed for the early warning signs section. If the person notices symptoms that indicate things are breaking down, like starting to spend excessive amounts of money, chain smoking or having more intense pain, the person follows the plan developed for "When Things Are Breaking Down."

If in a crisis situation, the plan will help the person discover that supporters should know they are needed. However, in certain crisis situations, the person may not be aware or willing to admit that he/she is in crisis. This is why having a strong team of supporters is so important. Supporters will observe the symptoms the person listed and take over responsibility for care, whether or not the person is willing to admit he/she is in a crisis at that time. Distributing the crisis plan to supporters and discussing it with them is absolutely essential to the person's safety and well-being.

HELPING OTHERS DEVELOP ACTION PLANS

If you are in a helping profession–a case manager, counselor, therapist, social worker, doctor–or even as a family member or friend, you can help support another person develop their personal action plan. You may do this with a group of people or with individuals. Whether you are working with individuals or groups, there are some general guidelines you need to follow. In addition, there are some specific strategies that will assist you in this work.

General Guidelines for Working with Individuals and Groups in Developing a WRAP

1. As a helper, you can make suggestions and share observations and ideas. Do not *require* anyone to do anything. Do not tell the person what to do or what to write. This would violate the basic premise that this action plan is developed by the person who will be using it. If you can't think of anything to say, just listen. Let the person or people know that that is what you are doing.
2. Avoid correcting spelling and grammar. These are not important in the planning process and might inhibit the person who is developing the plan.
3. Treat the person who is developing the plan with dignity, compassion, respect and unconditional high regard at all times.
4. Develop the plan at a pace that is comfortable for the individual who is developing the plan. Avoid setting rigid time schedules around development or completion of the plan. Some parts of the plan are difficult for people because they remind the person of hard times in the past or because the person may not have been aware of the "cause and effect" relationships between life circumstances and symptoms or hard times. The person should work on the plan only as long as the person feels comfortable. Then put it away for another time. For many people it is like discovering that the world is round and it takes some time to get used to the idea.
5. There is no right or wrong way to develop a plan unless it is injurious to the person–then it is wrong. People should feel free to customize the plan in any way that most effectively meets their needs. At the same time it is important to be realistic. People may have a hard time recognizing symptoms until they become very severe. If someone tries to tell you that pain so severe that he/she can't walk or being semi-conscious is an early warning sign, you can gently but firmly disagree and suggest it is a crisis situation.
6. Always give the person or people you are working with a message of hope. No one can predict the course of anyone else's illness or situation. Sometimes the most difficult cases turn out very well.
7. Encourage personal responsibility, and self advocacy.
8. Do not judge, criticize, blame or shame the person you are working with. This never helps and always makes it difficult for the person to have high self esteem, self advocate or take personal responsibility.

9. Use a tone of voice and body language that is encouraging and supportive. If your frustration and feelings of helplessness overwhelm you, shorten the session and set up another time to continue this work. Get some support for yourself. If working with this person or group of people is too hard for you, find someone else to take over.

10. If you are a health care provider, set up a relationship with the person you are working with that focuses on equality and mutuality, rather than on a hierarchical system where the health care provider is assumed to be the expert. Keep in mind that no one knows more about this situation, whatever it may be, than the person who is experiencing it.

Keep in mind that for many years, and particularly with certain types of illness or circumstances, there has been an implication that the individual has done something wrong or bad and is to blame for the illness or circumstance. Also, many treatments have been dehumanizing and blaming. The effects of all of this can devastate self esteem, and get in the way of healing and physical and emotional wellness. Your work is counteracting these devastating scenarios.

Working with Individuals

Many people like to have someone support them as they work on developing their action plans. If you are that support person, you can use the following steps as a guide in doing this work. If possible, have the person read through the directions for developing a Wellness Recovery Action Plan before you begin so both of you have a basic understanding of the task you are about to undertake and so the person will be clear about the benefits of following the plan.

Then begin by reviewing together some of the most common wellness tools. The person developing the plan makes a list (you could write it for the person if he/she has a difficult time writing) of those tools the person feels would be most useful. Then the two of you can brainstorm other possible tools–or things the person wants to avoid.

Then, using this list of tools as a reference point, work through the plan together section by section, beginning with the Daily Maintenance Plan, spending as much time as needed on each section. However, some people like to begin with the Crisis Plan and work back from there. Work sessions can be as long or as short as you and the person you are working with want them to be. Some people may choose not to develop a Crisis Plan or to leave it until another time. Whatever a person feels comfortable doing is the right thing to do.

Working with Groups on Developing Personal Action Plans

Developing Personal Action Plans is well suited to group work. I have worked with many groups, both large and small, in developing these plans. I begin by introducing participants to the planning process by going over each step–needed supplies, developing a Wellness Toolbox and a Daily Maintenance Plan, identifying triggers, early warning signs and those times when things are breaking down along with action plans for addressing these symptoms when they arise, and crisis planning.

Then I describe some of the most common tools or responses–sharing as much information on each of these tools as time allows. Then I ask the participants to share other tools that they have discovered, writing their responses on a sheet of newsprint. This sheet is then posted so participants can refer to it as they develop their plans.

Next I work with the group on each section of the plan–sharing common responses on each section, asking for their ideas and then writing them on newsprint for referral. If group members have their own supplies with them, they can work on their plan as ideas resonate with them. If possible I input the data on these sheets and give copies to each participant at the next meeting for easy referral. Someone in the group may be able to do this for you.

There are many benefits to the WRAP. It is a systematic method for developing skills in self-management and empowerment. It provides a means for individuals with a mental illness to work more collaboratively with health care providers. It is highly individualized and addressed the unique needs of the person and his/her situation. It is applicable to most any long-term illness/disability or problem situation. These benefits suggest that it can be used more widely and should be introduced as an option for individuals in need of a self-management system.

REFERENCES

Copeland, M.E. (1992). *The Depression Workbook: A Guide to Living with Depression and Manic Depression.* Oakland, CA: New Harbinger Publications.
Copeland, M.E. (1994). *Living Without Depression and Manic Depression: A Workbook for Maintaining Mood Stability.* Oakland, CA: New Harbinger Publications.

Copeland, M.E. (1994). *Strategies for Living with Depression and Manic Depression.* Audiotape. Oakland, CA: New Harbinger Publications.

Copeland, M.E. (1999). *Winning Against Relapse: A Workbook of Action Plans for Recurring Health and Emotional Problems.* Oakland, CA: New Harbinger Publications.

Copeland, M.E. (1999). *Winning Against Relapse.* Audiotape. Oakland, CA: New Harbinger Publications.

Copeland, M.E. (2000). *The Loneliness Workbook.* Oakland, CA: New Harbinger Publications.

Copeland, M.E. (2000). *Healing the Trauma of Abuse: A Women's Workbook.* Oakland, CA: New Harbinger Publications.

Copeland, M.E. (2000). *The Worry Control Workbook.* Oakland, CA: New Harbinger Publications.

Participatory Action Research:
A Model for Establishing Partnerships
Between Mental Health Researchers
and Persons with Psychiatric Disabilities

Melisa Rempfer, PhD
Jill Knott, MA

SUMMARY. Traditionally, mental health research has been conducted exclusively by professionals with little input and participation from individuals with mental illness themselves. Participatory action research (PAR) provides a more dynamic method of research, giving individuals the opportunity to become activists and advocates by influencing the direction of mental health research. This paper outlines important differences between PAR methodology and traditional research, with an emphasis on the differing roles of persons with mental illness in the two models. PAR is consistent with the recovery movement in several ways: both approaches value self-definition, empowerment, and experiential knowledge. As an example, this paper describes one project that incorporates principles of the participatory action research paradigm. *[Article copies available for a fee from The Haworth Document Delivery Service: 1-800-HAWORTH. E-mail address: <getinfo@haworthpressinc.com> Website: <http://www.HaworthPress.com> © 2001 by The Haworth Press, Inc. All rights reserved.]*

Melisa Rempfer and Jill Knott are affiliated with the University of Kansas Medical Center.

[Haworth co-indexing entry note]: "Participatory Action Research: A Model for Establishing Partnerships Between Mental Health Researchers and Persons with Psychiatric Disabilities." Rempfer, Melisa and Jill Knott. Co-published simultaneously in *Occupational Therapy in Mental Health* (The Haworth Press, Inc.) Vol. 17, No. 3/4, 2001, pp. 151-165; and: *Recovery and Wellness: Models of Hope and Empowerment for People with Mental Illness* (ed: Catana Brown) The Haworth Press, Inc., 2001, pp. 151-165. Single or multiple copies of this article are available for a fee from The Haworth Document Delivery Service [1-800-HAWORTH, 9:00 a.m. - 5:00 p.m. (EST). E-mail address: getinfo@haworthpressinc.com].

KEYWORDS. Participatory action research (PAR), psychiatric disabilities, recovery

As the principles of empowerment, inclusion and recovery have received increasing support in a variety of systems, Participatory action research (PAR) has emerged as an important approach to research and social change in disability and rehabilitation communities (Balcazar, Keys, Kaplan, & Suarez-Balcazar, 1998). PAR is a model of research in which the people under study (traditionally called "research subjects") actively participate with the professional researchers throughout the entire research process–from the initial conceptualization of the research, throughout its implementation, and even in the interpretation and presentation of findings (Danley & Ellison, 1999; White, Nary & Froehlich, 2001; Whyte, 1991).

PAR differs from traditional approaches to research methodology in several respects. One of the characteristic differences in PAR is the elevated role of the individuals in the community under study (White, Nary & Froehlich, 2001). In traditional research methods, the population under study is viewed as the passive "subject" of research, whereas research professionals are the "active" investigators who design and implement a study that attempts to minimize bias by keeping a neutral distance from the subjects. PAR, in contrast, demands that professional researchers engage *with* individuals who have a stake in the research. Traditionally, the role of "expert" is granted to the professional (in this example, the professional researcher); however, in PAR methodology, the stakeholders are elevated to the role of experts and co-researchers, while the professional researchers take on roles similar to research consultants, collaborators, or learners.

Participatory action research has its roots in the traditions of both "participatory research" and "action research." First, as discussed by Danley and Ellison (1999), participatory research approaches are based on the idea that relevant stakeholders must always participate in any research that attempts to study them. This participation by stakeholders is valued as a method of maximizing the meaningfulness of the research. For instance, if only professional researchers, or "outsiders," are involved in designing a research project and choosing the methods of evaluation, it is likely that these professionals will be unable to capture the most accurate information about the group they hope to study. Because professionals lack the firsthand experience to which the stakeholders are privy, their efforts may be misdirected at times.

Stakeholder or consumer participation, on the other hand, can shape the research questions and strategies in such a way to make them most relevant to the actual lived experiences of that particular group (Rogers & Palmer-Ebbs, 1994). In addition, participation by the relevant stakeholders can serve to strengthen the investment of the research subjects toward the researchers and the project itself (Danley & Ellison, 1999). The group or community under study will experience a greater commitment toward any research project if stakeholders or community members are included in the process. Clearly, any research project is strengthened when all parties are committed and invested in the process.

Participatory action research also grows out of the action research tradition (Danley & Ellison, 1999). Whereas some traditional research is concerned only with the generation of knowledge or theory, action research is more demanding–it requires that researchers also create change and improvements. Participatory action research, then, not only involves stakeholders in the process of research, it also helps to mobilize them toward some desired change, such as policy changes in a service system, or community health behavior changes. One primary goal of PAR is to directly impact and improve the lives of the individuals in the research. This goal is clearly a distinction between PAR and more traditional forms of research (Balcazar et al., 1998).

APPLYING PAR WITHIN A MENTAL HEALTH CONTEXT

The use of participatory research has primarily focused on individuals with physical disabilities (Balzacar et al., 1998; Campbell, Copeland, & Tate, 1998); however, the scope of the movement is evolving to include individuals with psychiatric disorders (Chamberlin & Rogers, 1990; Rogers & Palmer-Erbs, 1994). As is true with other applications of PAR, this paradigm applied to individuals with mental illness provides the opportunity for more relevant questions to be asked by those who have the most to gain from the research (Rogers & Palmer-Erbs, 1994). Thus, outcomes forged by this partnership could prove helpful in maximizing realistic changes in lives of people with psychiatric disabilities.

An important new emphasis in mental health services for individuals with psychiatric disabilities is the rise of community-based services. To varying degrees most community treatment centers focus on independent living within one's own community and therefore provide relevant tools, skills and resources for consumers. In accordance with the mission of community centers, PAR also supports this ideology. However, PAR moves beyond "traditional" practices and activities of community-based programs, by seeking to improve the shortcomings of traditional practices from the consumer's point of view. PAR approaches have the advantage of increasing the scope and relevance of research; consumer involvement can provide fresh perspectives that generate new ideas and develop solutions that increase consumer satisfaction.

Because mental health research traditionally defines persons with mental illness as "patients," there tends to be an even larger gap between professional researchers and research participants in this arena. Consequently, PAR may have particular relevance for consumers of mental health services who have been excluded from decision-making both in terms of research and clinical services. By including the voice of consumers with mental illness, researchers will be exposed to new ideas and perspectives that have not been represented in the professional and scientific literature to date. Furthermore, PAR provides a forum that is both supportive and respectful of consumer's abilities to identify and shape the type of research most meaningful for them. Within this setting, consumers can pose questions about research models, voice concerns about various theories or methods, and offer solutions consistent with their point of view. To this end, PAR focuses on power sharing, relationship building, and social changes, thus breaking down the traditional roles of "patient" versus "professional."

Another related aspect of PAR that merits attention is the potential to reduce social discrimination and prejudice regarding psychiatric disabilities. One may speculate that as professionals and consumer collaborators become equal partners in designing, implementing, and disseminating information, a beneficial effect may indirectly occur among the larger community. Therefore of special interest, is whether societal attitudes may begin to change as individuals with psychiatric disorders are viewed as equal, competent partners of "professionals," rather than a distinct or different sub-group of people. Therefore, one of the promising directions of PAR is to challenge and counteract the stigma and oppression often attached to those with psychiatric disabilities.

The emergence of PAR as a legitimate approach to mental health research is paralleled by the increasing prominence of self-help/mutual aid efforts. Self-help/mutual aid groups are "grass roots" organizations run by and for people with psychiatric disabilities. The main focus is to create social changes by adapting mental health services in ways that consumers feel are responsive to their needs. Thus, in many ways, participatory action research is consistent with the ideology and philosophy of self-help/mutual aid groups. Nelson et al. (1998) cited a slogan taken from a South African disability movement that captures the intent and spirit of mutual aid/self-help organizations: "Nothing about me, without me." Self-help/mutual aid groups are based on everyday lived experiences of their constituents, some focusing on political activism, and social change, others working to develop socially supportive groups (Nelson et al., 1998). Therefore, merging and respecting the recommendations of those involved in self-help/mutual aid would further identify important ideas and desired direction for change. Basing the "applied research" investigations of PAR upon the issues and recommendations made by self-help/mutual aid groups might strengthen arguments or lobbying efforts for substantive changes to be made in mental health legislation.

CHALLENGES TO PARTICIPATORY RESEARCH IN MENTAL HEALTH SETTINGS

One of the challenges PAR faces is the possibility that consumers who are most disenfranchised from professionals will not participate in research. PAR projects need to engage as many consumers as possible to be successful. Nonetheless, research and community support services are unable to attract a certain percentage of persons with mental illness. For instance, Anthony, Cohen, and Kennard (1990) suggest that a significant number of individuals with psychiatric disabilities choose not to affiliate with a community-based system because the services are "unappealing, inappropriate, or demeaning." Furthermore, they suggest non-participation is due to inadequacies of the system rather than the limitations or deficits of those with mental illness. With regard to PAR, it may be similarly true that some individuals will be less likely to participate with researchers in such efforts. PAR projects should be designed to maximize participation and researchers who engage in PAR should make efforts to engage people with a diversity of perspectives. Several strategies, including assertive outreach and flexibility, will assist in recruiting a broad base of participant involvement. Such efforts by professional researchers will improve the research by involving a more representative group of people with mental illness in the project. Relatedly, attempts to include traditionally excluded persons may prove beneficial at the individual level as well. For instance, individuals who participate in research and are respected and recognized as valuable

members of the process will likely feel an improved sense of empowerment, self-efficacy and hope. If PAR facilitates changes such as these, it
has served an important purpose.

Another challenge to PAR is familiarizing consumers with research
methods. Consumer collaborators will be called upon to evaluate and
resolve many questions or issues related to the research project, thus
PAR must focus on teaching consumers the fundamentals of research
design. PAR is a departure from traditional research in which individuals with psychiatric disabilities are "passive objects of study" (Balcazar
et al., 1998); these new members of the scientific teams are likely to feel
somewhat uncomfortable in their new roles. As discussed earlier, PAR
is designed to provide consumers with a sense of empowerment by
"gaining and increasing knowledge" (Nelson et al., 1998, p. 886). Thus
"knowledge" will validate their sense of equality. To this end, "professional" researchers should provide a creative learning environment, for
example workshops in formal and informal settings (Rogers &
Palmer-Erbs, 1994). The first strategy is that of conceptualizing the information. Initially, didactic aids such as examples of research drawn
from relevant designs, illustrating critical point can be presented in a
traditional "classroom" setting. A second strategy assumes that extensive practice is necessary to assimilate the information. Therefore,
within this context, manuals that outline and organize the content and
concepts presented during each lesson and include practice could be included. Consumers could then begin to generate alternative method-
ological strategies, thus encouraging problem solving, thinking and the
acquisition of knowledge by all parties.

Although it is important to recognized these potential challenges to
the use of PAR methods, we believe that the advantages of the approach
in mental health research far outweigh the difficulties. In fact, some of
the difficulties reflect the unique benefits of the PAR approach: namely,
the ability of participant-driven research to challenge the status quo.
Ideally, consumers involved in a PAR project express their ideas freely,
without fear of negative evaluation. Essentially, PAR approaches invite
changes within the current systems to ensure that consumers' voices are
heard. As Nelson et al. (1998) states, "Defining their own reality height-
ens consciousness, and participants may begin to challenge expert or
dominant ideas and empowerment is fostered." The most productive
and meaningful changes can arise from consumers whose ideas dissent
from current theories and practices.

PAR AND RECOVERY AS COMPATIBLE IDEALS

In recent years, there has been an increasing recognition that recovery from major mental illness is a realistic and important process (Deegan, 1997). Recovery can take on a variety of meanings, some of which are very personal and subjective. However, there are some basic themes that characterize the concept of recovery from serious mental illness, such as self-definition, empowerment, and a process-oriented approach (Deegan, 1997; Young & Ensing, 1999). It is easy to see that PAR and recovery share several common ideals.

Self-Definition

A core value that characterizes many discussions about recovery for people with psychiatric disabilities is the need for self-definition. Deegan (1997) has described how throughout history people have been marginalized and devalued by being placed in categories such as "*the* mentally ill" or "schizophrenic" and other psychiatric labels. Such terms are increasingly recognized as oppressive because they strip individuals of their personhood and instead identify them by a psychiatric label. Further, these psychiatric labels are not self-generated descriptors; they are categories constructed and used by the mental health system and society at large.

Among other things, recovery is about individuals defining for themselves how they choose to be seen. In terms of descriptors this might entail being seen as a "person with a psychiatric disability," "consumer," or "survivor," rather than "patient." And, likely, it might mean seeing oneself as a "student" or "mother" or "musician" well before any mental-health focused descriptor. By engaging in active self-definition, persons who traditionally have been labeled and seen as passive can begin to emerge as having more control over their own experiences and relationships with others. This is particularly true in relationships that traditionally have had such unequal power distributions, such as those between consumers and mental health professionals or researchers.

As with the recovery process, the success of PAR depends on the active self-definition of persons with psychiatric disabilities. In fact, research projects that follow PAR methodology are built *from the very start* on participant-driven definitions. PAR researchers start by asking the questions that arise from within the communities or individuals under study. Instead of the traditional research paradigm in which the researchers decide what is important to study, PAR approaches look to the individuals to define for themselves their strengths, needs or questions. As a research project progresses, researchers look to the participants for continual definitions or understanding from their own perspectives as individuals with psychiatric disabilities.

Empowerment

A second overlapping principle for recovery and PAR is the concept of empowerment. A fundamental aspect of PAR is that the professional researchers and the research participants share power and responsibility (Danley & Ellison, 1999). As a result, the professionals must relinquish some of the decision-making power they have traditionally held. Removing the power differential that traditionally exists between "professionals" and "research subjects" or "patients" is an essential aspect of any endeavor that purports to value either PAR or recovery.

Valuing the Process

Many who have discussed the concept of recovery for persons with psychiatric disabilities have described it as a journey or a process, rather that a particular end point or destination. In other words, recovery relates to an ongoing process of change, learning or healing. Similarly, PAR approaches value the process associated with learning just as much as the end product. In this regard, PAR approaches lend themselves to qualitative research and studies that focus on the *experience* of disability (Rogers & Palmer-Erbs, 1994).

In addition, PAR studies are often not over when the data are analyzed and research reports are written. Instead, PAR is seen as an ongoing process that will ultimately have an impact on communities or policies. Research stakeholders as well as professional researchers are seen as "change agents" (Rogers & Palmer-Erbs, 1994) extend their involvement beyond just the specific research project itself and into the realm of influencing policy, programs or communities.

PAR IN ACTION:
A SKILLS TRAINING PROJECT AS EXAMPLE

The preceding discussion highlights several values of the PAR methodology, but it is also important to understand how PAR might be brought to bear on a particular project. At the University of Kansas, we have been implementing a research project that utilizes PAR values and methods. At present, we are implementing a multi-site evaluation of a skills training program designed to improve grocery shopping skills. Our research program attempts to maximize the participation of persons with psychiatric disabilities and the sharing of power/authority among professional researchers and stakeholders. We recognize that PAR can be seen on a continuum and we are constantly exploring ways to maximize PAR in our work. We do not claim ours to be the only or even the best model of how to implement PAR with people who have psychiatric disabilities. However, we also recognize that presently the majority of research in the area of psychiatric disabilities is done without *any* meaningful participation or decision-making by stakeholders. Therefore, we hope that by describing the effect of PAR on our project, we can illustrate that it is a useful and realistic approach for research in the area of psychiatric disability. We will describe how we have attempted to incorporate PAR at various stages of our project, from the initial conceptualization, to planning and implementation, and, ultimately, to dissemination and promoting change.

Conceptualization of the project. As stated previously, an important aspect of PAR approaches is the inclusion of stakeholder participation at all phases of a project, including the initial conceptualization of research hypotheses, design or methodology. Our current project is built on prior work (e.g., Hamera & Brown, 2000) to examine outcome in terms of independent living skills for people with psychiatric disabilities. In order to determine which functional skills were of most relevance to people with psychiatric disabilities, Hamera and Brown (2000) interviewed consumers of local psychosocial and support programs and learned that many people found grocery shopping to be a particularly difficult task. Grocery shopping skills, therefore, became the initial starting point for future research in this area. Specifically, consumers identified the specific skill areas that we should address in an intervention/teaching program such as helping people identify lower priced grocery items. Focus groups were held throughout the pilot research projects to elicit participation and feedback from the research participants/stakeholders. Our current project, which examines the effectiveness of a grocery shopping skills training program, was largely shaped by this participant involvement throughout pilot work.

Planning the project. In planning the research design of this project, several key decisions were based on participant-stakeholder involvement. In addition to the feedback we elicited from research participants in the pilot phases of the research, we sought more extensive involve-

ment from individuals who agreed to participate in the planning and implementation of the current project. One aspect of this stakeholder
involvement includes the participation by Frederick Frese, PhD, as a
consultant to the project. With a unique voice as both a consumer and
mental health provider, Dr. Frese has spoken and written extensively
about recovery and consumer involvement in the mental health system
(e.g., Frese, 1998; Frese & Walker, 1997). In addition, the key project
staff includes several persons who are also consumers of mental health
services at the research sites. As project coordinators at their site, each
of these individuals work closely with other project staff and have been
involved in planning the specific research methodology.

One specific example of how consumer/stakeholder involvement has
influenced the project at the "planning" stage relates to the choices of
measures used in the study. Initial plans for the study included traditional measures (e.g., tests of cognition, symptoms, etc.), but did not adequately capture the strengths or positive qualities of our research
participants. By reminding us that so much psychiatric/mental health
research is deficit-focused, consumer/stakeholder involvement prompted
the inclusion in the study of an entire set of measures that emphasis positive qualities such as empowerment and hope (Rogers, Chamberlin,
Ellison, & Crean, 1997; Snyder et al., 1991). This aspect of our project
is much more consistent with a recovery focus.

Implementing the project. Throughout the actual research process,
consumer site coordinators will continue their involvement in significant ways. They will coordinate participant recruitment, conduct interviews with participants, and share responsibility with other staff members for conducting the skills training intervention group. The specific
duties will vary, depending on the skills and interests of each individual
consumer site coordinator. However, it is important to us that each
member of the research team be included in every possible aspect of the
project. Research team members will be encouraged to participate to
their fullest potential and choice.

Analysis, dissemination and change. Upon completion of the project
and data collection, PAR will be just as pivotal to this project as in earlier stages. We have described above the "participatory" aspect of PAR,
but the "action" is equally important. Consumers will continue to serve
as key project staff members throughout the final stages of the research
project. Their feedback regarding the social significance of the results
will inform the analysis and dissemination of the findings. To elicit further feedback about the findings, we plan to convene a series of meetings involving additional consumer/stakeholders and all project staff.

This group will together review and interpret the study's findings and make recommendations about relevant dissemination efforts and action plans. Dissemination efforts will include not only scientific outlets such as professional journals or meetings, but also dissemination to policy and consumer-oriented audiences. Certainly, by partnering with stake-holders/consumers/advocates we will be better suited to identify the full range of audiences.

Benefits and challenges. This description provides only a brief overview of our attempt to utilize a PAR approach in our current research project. The above-mentioned strategies will provide specific ways to infuse PAR into our work. We believe that all of these strategies will provide several overall benefits. First, because our research interests focus on community-based treatment models that increasingly are utilizing a recovery philosophy, the use of PAR methods is consistent with the research questions and the settings in which we work. As a result, we have found that our working relationships with these practice settings have been productive and cooperative. It is likely that another research model (i.e., one that maintains the traditional need for professional distance and "authority") would have distanced us further from the consumers, staff and administration at the community settings in which we choose to conduct our research. As more and more individuals with psychiatric disabilities live, work, and receive services within their own communities, it will be crucial that psychiatric research take place in those settings as well. In order to conduct this community-based research, it will become more incumbent upon investigators to conduct their science in ways that are congruent with the changing values of their constituents.

A second benefit of using PAR in our project has been that we have been held to a higher standard of accountability in our work. Not only are we responsible to all the traditional sources–granting agencies, academic administration, journal editors, etc.–but also to the consumers and even mental health professionals with whom we have partnered. For instance, because we attempt to communicate with team members using minimal jargon and unnecessary technical terms, we have been forced to clarify our thinking. As a result, we have become more disciplined about our scientific methods and choices.

A third major benefit with this approach has been that we are much better suited at logistical problem solving when we engage consumers and stakeholders in the decision-making process. Undoubtedly, problems and challenges will arise in any research project. As "outsider" researchers, it can be difficult to develop realistic solutions to logistical/planning difficulties such as recruitment problems, attrition from the study by participants, and scheduling or transportation obstacles. Because our research team includes members of the system/community under study, they are well-suited to generate potential solutions to such problems. Further, they are more likely to be successful in implementing these logistical solutions than we, as outsiders, have been.

Finally, perhaps the most personally rewarding benefit associated with the PAR approach is the renewed sense of enthusiasm that results from working together with our diverse and invested team. We are excited not only by the scientific aspects of our work, but PAR reminds us better than any other research methodology that the personal aspect is far more interesting. Through building personal relationships with our research partners, we find that our work has become more relevant, interesting, and enjoyable. Our own enthusiasm is equaled by that of the research team. Team members have reported on several occasions that they find great satisfaction by participating in a project they view as important and personally meaningful.

We have also found that PAR poses special challenges in this project. In fact, some of the benefits mentioned previously are, at times, challenging. One common challenge in PAR is the increased time and resource commitment involved when including team members with limited (or no) previous research experience. To address this issue we have held several full-day sessions to discuss research methods and to train team members on interviewing and other specific skills necessary for the project. Although this process is time-consuming, we have also found it to be an excellent opportunity for team building.

An additional caution for PAR researchers is to recognize that including persons with mental illness in the research process is not a panacea. We must constantly remind ourselves that even with participant representation, no research project can adequately capture the diverse perspectives or needs of all persons. Although we can (and do) make efforts to engage a variety of voices and opinions in a project, we must also recognize that none of us can truly speak for everyone. As such, PAR researchers must also exhibit caution and recognize the realistic limits of our conclusions.

FUTURE DIRECTIONS

We hope that sharing our experiences with participatory action research displays that it is a viable and beneficial approach to mental health research. Although it is not yet a common approach to research, there appears to be a growing appreciation for PAR as various stakeholders demand research that is meaningful, respectful and empowering. We believe that our own partnership with consumers produces rigorous research that reflects the issues most relevant to the actual experiences of persons with psychiatric disabilities.

Although some agencies and researchers have advocated the use of PAR, there is much more that needs to be done before it is likely to become a common practice. We propose several strategies that may promote PAR. First, although some funding agencies have supported and encouraged PAR methodology (e.g., NIDRR), more research agencies should follow this lead and explicitly support, or even mandate, research that includes stakeholder participation. Surely, this is one effective way for researchers to become aware of and motivated toward PAR strategies. Second, graduate and other research training should begin to address PAR approaches to scientific research. PAR methods will certainly increase in popularity if new generations of researchers are exposed to its benefits and taught the methods during their training.

But the burden lies not only with the scientific community. It is our hope that increasingly, consumers, advocacy organizations, and mental health systems will embrace (and demand) the use of PAR. By their active participation with universities and researchers, these individuals and agencies can contribute to the generation of more relevant, empowering, and respectful research projects and ultimately, social change.

ACKNOWLEDGMENTS

We are fortunate to work with many individuals whose ideas and effort have contributed to our experience of PAR. To our colleagues at the University of Kansas Medical Center, Tana Brown, PhD, OTR, and Edna Hamera, PhD, ARNP, we owe many thanks for your collaboration on this and other projects. We extend a special thanks to Dr. Frederick Frese for his support and feedback, which has influenced us in many ways. Finally, we wish to acknowledge several members of our research team: Scott Hess, Amy Peterson, Laura Harper, Monica Welch, Joe Thorne, Kathy Campbell, Frank Findling, and Jason Wollenberg. Thank you for your commitment and partnerships.

We gratefully acknowledge support from the National Institute on Disability and Rehabilitation Research (grant # H133G000152).

REFERENCES

Anthony, W. A., Cohen, M., & Kennard, W. (1990). Understanding the current facts and principles of mental health systems planning. *American Psychologist, 45* (11), 1249-1252.

Balcazar, B.E., Keys, C.B., Kaplan, D.L., & Suarez-Balcazar, Y. (1998). Participatory action research and people with disabilities: Principles and challenges. *Canadian Journal of Rehabilitation, 12*(2), 105-112.

Campbell, M., Copeland, B., & Tate, B. (1998). Taking the standpoint of people with disabilities in research: Experiences with participation. *Canadian Journal of Rehabilitation, 12*(2), 95-104.

Chamberlin, J., & Rogers, J. A. (1990). Planning a community-based mental health system. Perspective of service recipients. *American Psychologist, 45*(11), 1241-1244.

Danley, K. & Ellison, M. L. (1999). *A Handbook for Participatory Action Researchers.* (Available from the Center for Psychiatric Rehabilitation, Sargent College of Health and Rehabilitation Sciences, Boston University, 940 Commonwealth Avenue West, Boston, MA 02215).

Deegan, P.E. (1997) Recovery and empowerment for people with psychiatric disbalities. *Social Work in Health Care, 25*(3), 11-24.

Frese, F.J. (1997) The consumer-survivor movement, recovery, and consumer-professionals. *Professional Psychology: Research and Practice, 28*(3), 243-245.

Frese, F.J. & Davis, W.W. (1998) Advocacy, recovery, and the challenges of consumerism for schizophrenia. *Psychiatric Clinics of North America, 21*(1), 233-249.

Hamera, E. & Brown, C.E. (2000). Developing a context-based performance measure for persons with schizophrenia: The Test of Grocery Shopping Skills. *American Journal of Occupational Therapy Education, 54*(1), 20-25.

Nelson, G., Ochocka, J., Griffin, K., & Lord, J. (1998). "Nothing about me, without me": Participatory action research with self-help/mutual aid organizations for psychiatric consumers/survivors. *American Journal of Community Psychology, 26*(6), 881-912

Rappaport, J. (1993). Narrative studies, personal stories, and identity transformation in the mutual help context. *The Journal of Applied Behavioral Science, 29*(2), 239-256.

Rogers, E.S., & Palmer-Erbs, V. (1994). Participatory action research: Implications for research and evaluation in psychiatric rehabilitation. *Psychosocial Rehabilitation Journal, 18*(2), 3-12

Rogers, S.E., Chamberlin, J., Ellison, M.L. & Crean, T. (1997). A consumer-constructed scale to measure empowerment among users of mental health services. *Psychiatric Services, 48*(8), 1042-1047.

Snyder, C. R., Harris, C., Anderson, J. R., Holleran, S. A., Irving, L. M., Sigmon, S. T., Yoshinobu, L., Gibb, J., Langelle, C., & Harney, P. (1991). The will and the ways: Development and validation of an individual differences measure of hope. *Journal of Personality and Social Psychology, 60,* 570-585.

White, G.W., Nary, D.E., & Froehlich, A.K. (2001). Consumers as collaborators in research and action. *Journal of Prevention & Intervention in the Community, 21,* 15-34.

Whyte, W.F. (1997). *Participatory Action Research.* Thousand Oaks, CA: Sage Publications.

Young, S.L., & Ensing, D.S. (1999). Exploring recovery from the perspective of people with psychiatric disabilities. *Psychiatric Rehabilitation, 22*(3), 219-231.

Index

Accommodations, 33, 51
Adult Sensory Profile,
     106,115-116,120-121,124
African Americans, misdiagnosis of,
     68-69
Americans with Disabilities Act,
     16,33,50
Angry indignation, 10

Carr, Vaughn, 19
Clay, Sally, 67
Colorado State University, 49
Confidentiality, 32
Consumer provider, 24,33-36,40-41,
     55-56
Consumers as Providers Training
     Program, 38,55-57
Crisis planning, 145-152
Critical consciousness, 90-91

Daily maintenance list, 129,132-134
Dehumanization, 9-10
Diagnosis of mental illness,
     7-9,19,25,45,65,71-72
Diagnostic and Statistical Manual (of
     Mental Disorders), 9,65,69
Doolittle, Hilda, 75-76
Dreams, 10-11,24,40-41,99
Drop in center, 28-30
Dunn's model of sensory processing,
     115-121,123

Early warning signs, 129,135-137
Eliot, T.S., 75

Empowerment, 27,29,106-107,109,113,
     117,158
Executive approach to teaching, 85-87
Evidence for recovery, 19-20

First National Forum on Recovery from
     Mental Illness, 67
Frese, Frederick, 65,73,160
Freud, Sigmund, 68,75

Hearing Voices Network, 76-77
Hope, hopelessness, 10-11,24,35,37
Hospitalization, 8,25-26,47-48,99
Humanist psychology, 88

Jamison, Kay Redfield, 74-75
Johnson County Mental Health Center, 31
Journey of Hope, 37

Kansas Mental Health Reform Act, 27-28
Kraepelin, Emil, 10

Lauper, Cyndi, 57
Lawrence, D.H., 75
Level II Fieldwork, 51,98,113
Liberationist approach to teaching,
     89-93

Mirrors of Madness, 62
Moeller, Mary, 56
Mudrow, John, 66

   167

T - #0556 - 101024 - C0 - 212/152/10 - PB - 9780789019059 - Gloss Lamination